Sudden Sensorineural Hearing Loss

Guillermo Plaza
José Ramón García Berrocal
Editors

Sudden Sensorineural Hearing Loss

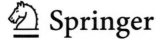 Springer

Editors
Guillermo Plaza
Ear, Nose and Throat Department
Hospital Universitario de Fuenlabrada
Madrid, Spain

Ear, Nose and Throat Department
Hospital Universitario Sanitas La Zarzuela
Madrid, Spain

Universidad Rey Juan Carlos
Madrid, Spain

José Ramón García Berrocal
Ear, Nose and Throat Department
Hospital Universitario Puerto de Hierro
Majadahonda, Madrid, Spain

Universidad Autónoma de Madrid
Madrid, Spain

ISBN 978-3-031-61384-5   ISBN 978-3-031-61385-2   (eBook)
https://doi.org/10.1007/978-3-031-61385-2

Translation from the Spanish language edition: "Sordera Súbita" by Guillermo Plaza and José Ramón García Berrocal, © Guillermo Plaza, José Ramón García Berrocal 2022. Published by Ergon, Madrid, Barcelona. All Rights Reserved.

This Springer imprint is published by the registered company Springer Nature Switzerland AG
The registered company address is: Gewerbestrasse 11, 6330 Cham, Switzerland

If disposing of this product, please recycle the paper.

To my wife, Araceli, for her unconditional love. To Pepe and Concha, my dedicated and tireless proofreaders. To my parents, always present.

To my colleagues at Hospital Universitario de Fuenlabrada and Hospital Universitario La Zarzuela, for their dedication to daily care work.

To patients suffering from sudden sensorineural hearing loss, in the hope of achieving more effective treatments for them in the future.

GUILLERMO

To my family and especially to María Jesús, for her eternal support and endless patience.

To all my colleagues who have been involved with this exciting project launched more than 30 years ago.

To patients with sudden sensorineural hearing loss for their invaluable participation that will help us manage their condition better.

JOSÉ RAMÓN

Foreword

It gives me great pleasure to write this foreword for Dr. Guillermo Plaza and Dr. Jose Ramon Garcia Berrocal's English language Handbook on *Sudden Sensorineural Hearing Loss*. I have read their previous work over many years and the original Spanish language book and handbook, and I am glad that the world of otolaryngologists and audiologists who do not read Spanish fluently will now be able to learn from these masters.

This is called a Basic Handbook, but it is a thorough compilation of the information that is known about diagnosis, possible etiologies, and possible treatments for sudden sensorineural hearing loss (SSNHL). The collection of 11 chapters in this Handbook allows for concise but detailed understanding of each subject within SSNHL, with a view to future developments that we, as treating physicians, audiologists, and researchers, should look for.

One of the things about SSNHL which I find somewhat unique in Otolaryngology is the ease with which information has been shared across continents, countries, and cultures, in order to benefit the most patients. To that end, I will reiterate what one of our colleagues in Sao Paulo, Brasil, Dra. Norma de Oliveira Penido, has highlighted. SSNHL is not a disease. It is a symptom. The underlying pathology causing this alarming loss of a vital sense is often not known, particularly at the onset. As we look at treatments that work well or poorly, it is important to keep in mind that we are offering medicine or hyperbaric oxygen or possible other treatments for a *symptom* without knowing the underlying *disease*. It is important that we understand this conundrum and that we explain it to our patients and their families, so that we can keep high but realistic expectations for return of hearing, diminution of tinnitus, and restoration of quality of life. This lends itself well to shared decision-making.

At the House Ear Institute in California, USA, under the leadership of Dr. William Slattery, the Hearing Science Accelerator has taken on the project of SSNHL, ensuring broad input from all stakeholders. Although in its initial stages, important information and meaningful pathways for diagnosis, research, and treatment have been identified. The Brasilian team, led by Dra. Penido, is showing us the utility of extended high-frequency audiometry as well as assessment of depression and anxiety, in the management of these patients. This, and the work of Drs. Plaza and García Berrocal, speaks to the high level of international collaboration and idea exchange in SSNHL.

As we wrote the American Academy of Otolaryngology-*Head and Neck Surgery's Clinical Practice Guideline on Sudden Hearing Loss* in 2012 and the Update in 2019, we identified current practices that work, current practices that do not work, and areas where research is urgently needed. Researchers from around the world heeded that information, and Drs. Plaza and García Berrocal's Handbook showcases the new material as well as the more established protocols. Authorship of this Handbook includes otolaryngologists, audiologists, radiologists, and other professionals involved in the care of these patients. It is beautifully collated and will be a great asset for those interested in the evidence-based care of these patients.

American Otological Society   Sujana S. Chandrasekhar
St Petersburg, FL, USA

American Academy of Otolaryngology-Head
and Neck Surgery
Alexandria, VA, USA

ENT and Allergy Associates, LLP
New York, NY, USA

Department of Otolaryngology-Head
and Neck Surgery
Zucker School of Medicine at Northwell
Hempstead, NY, USA

Prologue

It is an honour and a pleasure that the editors asked me to write the prologue to this handbook on sudden sensorineural hearing loss, a condition that has always interested me from both a clinical and a research point of view.

To date, the pathogenesis of idiopathic sudden sensorineural hearing loss (ISSNHL), its different clinical forms, prognostic factors, and optimal treatments are still an active field of research and subject of debate and controversy. Although years ago there was an unclear definition of this condition, today we at least have a specific concept that is applied universally.

ISSNHL is clinically characterised by rapid onset sensorineural hearing loss—in less than 3 days—of greater than 30 dB in at least three contiguous frequencies in pure tone audiometry without a known cause. After appropriate diagnostic study, less than a quarter of cases of sudden sensorineural hearing loss can be attributed to identifiable causes such as viruses, including several cases recently related to COVID-19 infection, vestibular schwannomas, inner ear haemorrhage, internal auditory canal metastasis, rupture of dermoid or toxic cysts, or noise, among others.

Although several years ago it was cited that the incidence of ISSNHL did not usually exceed 20 per 100,000 people per year, this incidence is not true at present. We have seen that it is increasing considerably due to increased risk factors and an ageing society. In addition, the above figures did not account for cases of spontaneous recovery that did not receive medical assistance. And of course, the current improvement in healthcare access and a better understanding of this entity are favouring a greater diagnosis.

It affects any age group, although mainly patients between 40 and 60 years old. It is rare in children. Spontaneous untreated recovery typically occurs within the first 2 weeks and in at least one-third of cases. Simultaneous bilateral involvement is rare.

A third of the cases of ISSNHL can be considered profound, affecting the patient both psychologically and socially. It can be associated with tinnitus and vertigo, thereby increasing the patient's disability and worsening the prognosis of hearing recovery, as the aggression to the inner ear in these cases is greater.

Dr Guillermo Plaza is an expert and enthusiastic researcher in the subject, with the scientific and leadership requirements to publish in a monograph on sudden sensorineural hearing loss in 2018, of which he was also the author. In this publication, prepared in cooperation with a group of experienced collaborators, we have compiled all the scientifically proven knowledge to date. Dr José Ramón García Berrocal is a clinical-experimental researcher specialised in the field of autoimmunity of the inner ear and sudden sensorineural hearing loss.

It is to these two professionals that we owe the publication of this handbook which, in my opinion, constitutes an excellent idea as it is a pathology that is consulted especially in the emergency department and which requires early diagnostic and therapeutic management. This handbook, an updated summary of the monograph, is very well organised and sets out to be a refresher of all the basics related to ISSNHL, the prognosis of which will depend hugely on how it is approached.

The support of Dr Guillermo Plaza from the Audiology Commission, and especially from Dr Mª José Lavilla, led to the creation of a register for ISSNHL patients, in which most hospitals in Spain now participate. This database is of huge interest not just epidemiologically but also to learn more about this condition and its response to different treatments. It therefore forms part of the first chapter of this handbook.

ISSNHL is primarily characterised by hypoxia in the inner ear and although its pathophysiology remains unknown, multiple associated underlying conditions such as viral infections, vascular occlusion, labyrinthine membrane ruptures, and autoimmune factors are assumed to be involved. The following two chapters use the authors' own research and other current projects to review the complexity of the possible mechanisms that trigger hearing loss.

The starting point of the diagnosis is to differentiate sensorineural hearing loss from conductive hearing loss. Special emphasis should be given to the collection of clinical data on medical history, risk factors, and previous conditions, to the basic physical examination (mainly otoscopy and acoumetry), and to the confirmation by pure tone and speech audiometry of its sensorineural origin. These aspects, as well as the usefulness of other complementary evidence, are discussed in their respective chapter.

The evolution of hearing recovery in ISSNHL is unpredictable as the underlying pathogenesis is variable. Prognostic factors of hearing recovery include age, severity of hearing loss, the audiogram, the presence of vertigo or tinnitus, associated metabolic disturbances, degree of hearing in the unaffected ear, and delay in treatment time.

We believe that there are still at least two key points for further progress in this regard. The first is to standardise the criteria of hearing recovery to homogenise results. The second involves the implementation of indications, start time, type, and optimal treatment dose for each specific case.

Although the therapeutic options offered over the years for ISSNHL have been innumerable, several chapters of this handbook present the treatments in which systematic reviews, quality clinical trials, clinical guides, and expert consensus provide greater effectiveness in hearing recovery. What most experts agree on is the importance of the early initiation of treatment. According to the recommended guidelines for the treatment of hearing loss in the AAO-HNS Clinical Guidance on ISSNHL, updated in 2019, steroid and hyperbaric oxygen therapy are the first options; always taking into account the doctor's judgement and the patient's preference. The use of intratympanic corticosteroids, either at onset or as salvage treatment, is increasingly widespread and supported in studies allowing for a higher concentration of the drug directly to the cochlea and without systemic effects. Treatment with hyperbaric oxygen depends on the availability of access to it, and its association with corticosteroids has obtained the best hearing recovery in the most recent studies.

Progress continues to be made and evidence is being provided on cellular and molecular levels, which may indicate the best treatment in the future. At present, however, we tend towards the personalised indication of an implantable device when there is no complete response with the usual treatments and when hearing loss is not sufficiently palliated with hearing aids. We conclude this handbook by providing references from expert surgeons on the benefit of different hearing implants in the treatment of patients with severe irreversible hearing loss due to ISSNHL.

In short, this handbook on ISSNHL fulfils its main objective of informing professionals who care for, diagnose, or treat these patients based on the most current evidence available. We believe that it is particularly recommended for frontline doctors, primary care ENT specialists, and family doctors.

Ear, Nose and Throat Department   Ana Maria García Arumí
Hospital Vall d'Hebron
Barcelona, Spain

Faculty of Medicine and Psychology
Universidad Autónoma de Barcelona
Barcelona, Spain

Preface

This manual, *Sudden Sensorineural Hearing Loss: A Basic Handbook* sets out to make one of the most frequent pathological entities of otological emergencies accessible to all doctors involved in its early diagnosis—principally family doctors and ENT specialists. To this end, the latest knowledge has been summarised in just ten chapters, which address different aspects such as epidemiology (chapter "Concept and Epidemiology of Sudden Sensorineural Hearing Loss"), aetiology (chapters "Aetiology of Sudden Sensorineural Hearing Loss: Autoimmune Hypothesis" and "Aetiology of Sudden Sensorineural Hearing Loss: Vascular, Viral or due to Perilymphatic Fistula"), diagnosis (chapters "Diagnostic Assessment and Complementary Tests in Sudden Sensorineural Hearing Loss" and "MRI in Sudden Sensorineural Hearing"), prognostic factors and analysis of results (chapter "Prognostic Factors and Recovery Criteria in Sudden Sensorineural Hearing Loss"), medical treatment (chapters "Treatment of Idiopathic Sudden Sensorineural Hearing Loss with Systemic Corticosteroids", "Treatment of Idiopathic Sudden Sensorineural Hearing Loss with Intratympanic Corticosteroids", and "Treatment of Sudden Sensorineural Hearing Loss with Hyperbaric Oxygen Therapy") and rehabilitative treatment using different hearing aids (chapter "Single-Sided Deafness (SSD) Hearing Aids: Airway Hearing Aids, Bone Conduction Hearing Aids, and Cochlear Implant Electrical Stimulation").

The aspects covered have drawn on the knowledge of various experts, most of whom have worked on the subject since the first meeting held in Madrid in 2009 that set out to achieve a consensus on the management of this condition from a nation-wide perspective. The aim was to unify criteria in the aspects studied and to respond to the many specialists who called for uniformity.

This handbook provides a logical evolution in the approach towards the topics, incorporating the latest technologies and diagnostic resources available, as well as modifying some of the diagnostic criteria and assessments of results in order to simplify and update the study of sudden sensorineural hearing loss. This ever-changing mindset demonstrates the authors' ability to take on the much-needed scientific perspective in the activity of the medical profession.

We are very honoured to be able to present this work in English, after its publication in Spanish in 2022. This has been possible, thanks to the generous help of our Editorial teams in Ergon and Springer.

Finally, we also want to thank all the authors for their generous availability and for their dedication in an era as committed to care as today's, which conditions much of our activity towards care and, therefore, limits our teaching and research work.

Madrid, Spain   Guillermo Plaza
Madrid, Spain   José Ramón García Berrocal

Acknowledgments

To Juan Medino and Montserrat Domínguez, of the library of the Hospital Universitario de Fuenlabrada.

Contents

Contributors

Marta Alcaraz Fuentes Ear, Nose and Throat Department, Hospital Universitario Sanitas La Zarzuela, Madrid, Spain

María Aragonés Redó Ear, Nose and Throat Department, Hospital Clínic Universitari de València, Valencia, Spain

Agustina Arbía Kalutich Ear, Nose and Throat Department, Hospital Universitario de Fuenlabrada, Madrid, Spain

Nuria Arnáiz Canora Ear, Nose and Throat Department, Hospital Universitario Puerto de Hierro, Majadahonda, Madrid, Spain

Felipe Benjumea Flores Ear, Nose and Throat Department, Hospitales Quirónsalud Marbella and Campo de Gibraltar, Cádiz, Spain

Juan Carlos Casado Morente Ear, Nose and Throat Department, Hospitales Quirónsalud Marbella and Campo de Gibraltar, Cádiz, Spain

Jordi Desola Alà Centro de Recuperación e Investigaciones Submarinas—Unidad de Terapia Hiperbárica (CRIS-UTH) [Centre for Underwater Recovery and Research—Hyperbaric Therapy Unit], Hospital Moisès Broggi, Sant Joan Despí, Barcelona, Spain

Hyperbaric Medicine at the Universidad de Barcelona, Barcelona, Spain

Ana María García Arumí Ear, Nose and Throat Department, Hospital Vall d'Hebron, Barcelona, Spain

Faculty of Medicine and Psychology, Universidad Autónoma de Barcelona, Barcelona, Spain

José Ramón García Berrocal Ear, Nose and Throat Department, Hospital Universitario Puerto de Hierro, Majadahonda, Madrid, Spain

Universidad Autónoma de Madrid, Madrid, Spain

Cristina García García Ear, Nose and Throat Department, Hospital Universitario de Fuenlabrada, Madrid, Spain

Ana Hernando García Diagnostic Imaging Department, Hospital Universitario de Fuenlabrada, Madrid, Spain

Mayte Herrera Ear, Nose and Throat Department, Hospital Universitario de Fuenlabrada, Madrid, Spain

Ear, Nose and Throat Department, Hospital Universitario Sanitas La Zarzuela, Madrid, Spain

Antonio Lara Peinado Ear, Nose and Throat Department, Hospital Universitario Sanitas La Zarzuela, Madrid, Spain

María José Lavilla Martín de Valmaseda Ear, Nose and Throat Department, Hospital Universitario Lozano Blesa, Zaragoza, Spain

Universidad de Zaragoza, Zaragoza, Spain

David R. Lobo Duro Ear, Nose and Throat Department, Hospital Universitario Marqués de Valdecilla, Santander, Cantabria, Spain

Valdecilla Biomedical Research Institute, Santander, Cantabria, Spain

Paula López Mesa Ear, Nose and Throat Department, Hospital Vall d'Hebron, Barcelona, Spain

Jaime Marco Algarra Ear, Nose and Throat Department, Hospital Clínic Universitari de València, Valencia, Spain

Universidad de Valencia, Valencia, Spain

Mar Martínez Ruiz-Coello Ear, Nose and Throat Department, Hospital Universitario de Fuenlabrada, Madrid, Spain

Estefanía Miranda Sánchez Ear, Nose and Throat Department, Hospital Universitario de Fuenlabrada, Madrid, Spain

Carmelo Morales Angulo Ear, Nose and Throat Department, Hospital Universitario Marqués de Valdecilla, Santander, Cantabria, Spain

Universidad de Cantabria, Santander, Cantabria, Spain

Juan José Navarro Sampedro Ear, Nose and Throat Department, Hospital Universitario de Donostia, Donostia-San Sebastián, Basque Country, Spain

Ear, Nose and Throat Department, Hospital Universitario de Donostia, Donostia-San Sebastián, Gipuzkoa, Spain

Carlos O'Connor-Reina Ear, Nose and Throat Department, Hospitales Quirónsalud Marbella and Campo de Gibraltar, Cádiz, Spain

Pablo Parente Arias Ear, Nose and Throat Department, Hospital Universitario A Coruña, A Coruña, Spain

Tomàs Pérez Carbonell Ear, Nose and Throat Department, Hospital Clínic Universitari de València, Valencia, Spain

Ignacio Pla Gil Ear, Nose and Throat Department, Hospital Clínic Universitari de València, Valencia, Spain

Guillermo Plaza Ear, Nose and Throat Department, Hospital Universitario de Fuenlabrada, Madrid, Spain

Ear, Nose and Throat Department, Hospital Universitario Sanitas La Zarzuela, Madrid, Spain

Universidad Rey Juan Carlos, Madrid, Spain

María Pujol Rodríguez Ear, Nose and Throat Department, Hospital Vall d'Hebron, Barcelona, Spain

Laura Rodríguez-Alcalá Ear, Nose and Throat Department, Hospitales Quirónsalud Marbella and Campo de Gibraltar, Cádiz, Spain

Concepción Rodríguez Izquierdo Ear, Nose and Throat Department, Hospital Universitario de Fuenlabrada, Madrid, Spain

Antonio Rodríguez Valiente Ear, Nose and Throat Department, Hospital Universitario Puerto de Hierro, Majadahonda, Madrid, Spain

Ana Sánchez Martínez Ear, Nose and Throat Department, Hospital Universitario Puerto de Hierro, Majadahonda, Madrid, Spain

Almudena Trinidad Cabezas Ear, Nose and Throat Department, Hospital Universitario Puerto de Hierro, Majadahonda, Madrid, Spain

Universidad Autónoma de Madrid, Madrid, Spain

María Urbasos Pascual Diagnostic Imaging Department, Hospital Universitario de Fuenlabrada, Madrid, Spain

Concept and Epidemiology of Sudden Sensorineural Hearing Loss

María José Lavilla Martín de Valmaseda,
Carmelo Morales Angulo, Pablo Parente Arias,
and Guillermo Plaza

Concept

Sudden sensorineural hearing loss (SSNHL), whether partial or total, unilateral or bilateral, is a condition which occurs suddenly and without a clear trigger [1–3]. It can be accompanied by symptoms of dizziness or may be isolated. When a cause of SSNHL is not observed, it is defined as idiopathic SSNHL (ISSNHL).

According to published consensus [2, 3], there are diagnostic criteria necessary for the diagnosis of SSNHL: (a) it is a sensorineural hearing loss greater than 30 dB; (b) it affects three or more consecutive frequencies; and (c) it occurs in <72 h. SSNHL can occur both in individuals with normal hearing and in individuals with prior sensorineural hearing loss.

M. J. Lavilla Martín de Valmaseda
Ear, Nose and Throat Department, Hospital Universitario Lozano Blesa, Zaragoza, Spain

Universidad de Zaragoza, Zaragoza, Spain

C. Morales Angulo
Ear, Nose and Throat Department, Hospital Universitario Marqués de Valdecilla, Santander, Cantabria, Spain

Universidad de Cantabria, Santander, Cantabria, Spain

P. Parente Arias
Ear, Nose and Throat Department, Hospital Universitario A Coruña, A Coruña, Spain

G. Plaza (✉)
Ear, Nose and Throat Department, Hospital Universitario de Fuenlabrada, Madrid, Spain

Ear, Nose and Throat Department, Hospital Universitario Sanitas La Zarzuela, Madrid, Spain

Universidad Rey Juan Carlos, Madrid, Spain
e-mail: guillermo.plaza@salud.madrid.org

© The Author(s), under exclusive license to Springer Nature Switzerland AG 2024
G. Plaza, J. R. García Berrocal (eds.), *Sudden Sensorineural Hearing Loss*,
https://doi.org/10.1007/978-3-031-61385-2_1

Table 1 Comparison of definitions of sudden sensorineural hearing loss (SSNHL)

Sudden sensorineural hearing loss	Idiopathic sudden sensorineural hearing loss	Probable sudden sensorineural hearing loss
Sensorineural hearing loss greater than 30 dB	Sensorineural hearing loss greater than 30 dB	Sensorineural hearing loss >10–20 dB
In three or more consecutive frequencies	In three or more consecutive frequencies	Affects two or three consecutive frequencies
Onset in <72 h	Onset in <72 h	Onset in <12 h
	Exclusion diagnosis after ruling out other aetiologies	

Meanwhile, *probable SSNHL* is defined as sensorineural or perceptual hearing loss in which only two or three frequencies are affected, with losses of 10–20 dB, appearing in <12 h. This definition includes hearing losses typically noted by the patient when they wake up in the morning, from which they recover quickly [4].

Despite the establishment of concise diagnostic criteria for SSNHL, it may be difficult to make the differential diagnosis with idiopathic fluctuating hearing losses, dilated vestibular aqueduct syndrome or, especially, Ménière's disease, as these conditions may meet these criteria at the beginning of the symptoms, without being the condition in question.

The different definitions of SSNHL are compared in Table 1.

For the diagnosis of SSNHL, it is necessary to first rule out any otological condition which justifies hearing loss [5]. For this, it is essential to perform an otoscopy that may show an organic cause of the hearing loss, such as wax or otitis media. In turn, acoumetry is very useful in clinical practice when making a differential diagnosis with a conductive hearing loss where findings with tuning forks are different from those expected in SSNHL.

However, it is pure tone audiometry that will provide us with the diagnosis of sensorineural hearing loss. If the patient has had a previous audiogram, this will be used as a reference when assessing the hearing loss that has occurred. If there are no previous audiometry exams, the healthy ear should be used as a reference [2].

Meanwhile, speech audiometry is gaining ground in the diagnosis and monitoring of the auditory evolution of SSNHL as it is more representative of the disability that this implies for the patient in their daily life [3, 6].

There are different clinical forms in which SSNHL occurs, depending on the frequencies affected by the hearing deficit (Fig. 1) [1]:

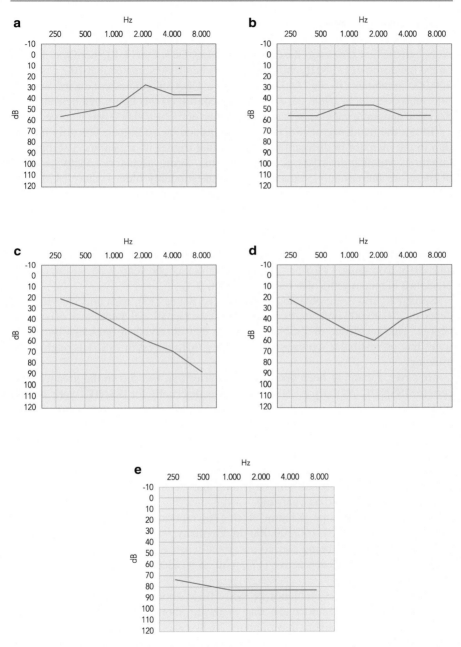

Fig. 1 Types of audiometric curves of sudden sensorineural hearing loss from the "Consensus on Diagnosis and Treatment of Sudden Sensorineural Hearing Loss" [1]. (**a**) Sudden sensorineural hearing loss (SSNHL) in low frequencies (usually related to a better prognosis). (**b**) Pantonal sudden sensorineural hearing loss. (**c**) Pantonal sudden sensorineural hearing loss in high frequencies. (**d**) Pantonal sudden sensorineural hearing loss in medium frequencies. (**e**) Profound sudden sensorineural hearing loss without functional hearing (cophosis)

Epidemiology

Although the first series was described in 1944 by De Kleyn [7, 8], there was no data on the incidence of ISSNHL until years later when Byl estimated it at 10.7 cases per 100,000 inhabitants in the Oakland area (CA, USA) in studies conducted in 1973 [9]. Subsequently, in 1984, the same author confirmed this figure in a new study in the same geographical area, where an incidence of 5–20/100,000 was recorded [10].

Today, the incidence of ISSNHL is perhaps somewhat higher, probably in relation to the increase in different risk factors that trigger its appearance: respiratory infections, vascular disorders, acoustic neuroma, cardiovascular risk factors, etc. All of these are increasingly frequent in an unquestionably older society [8, 11]. In addition, a better understanding of the condition, society's awareness and the improvement of accessibility to healthcare has also made this condition more diagnosed.

A recent study [12], which covers almost the entire population of South Korea, recorded a highly comprehensive study of the incidence of ISSNHL between 2011 and 2015, averaging 17.76 per 100,000 inhabitants per year, with an increase in incidence in recent years also being observed.

Similar figures were obtained in the United States [13], with an ISSNHL incidence of 27/100,000 inhabitants per year, based on a national database of 60 million people. This incidence of ISSNHL is twice that observed in otosclerosis and 20 times that of vestibular schwannoma, showing that interest in ISSNHL ought to be growing.

However, Japan has been one of the countries that has shown the greatest concern for ISSNHL. As early as 1973, the diagnostic criteria for ISSNHL were defined through a committee known as *Japan's Sudden Deafness Research Committee* [14]. Following these criteria, Kitaoku et al. [15] described the incidence of ISSNHL in the Japanese province of Nara in 1992–1993 as 18–21 cases per 100,000 inhabitants per year, although in some cities it reached up to 61 cases per 100,000 inhabitants per year. As a result, the implementation of these criteria led to a sustained increase in the incidence of this condition, confirming that it is more frequent in middle-aged patients between 45 and 65 years old.

Meanwhile, in Europe, Klemm et al. [16] reported in 2009 an incidence of ISSNHL of up to 100–160/100,000 in Germany, especially in regions where ISSNHL studies were being carried out. Finally, since 2000 the Swedish National ISSNHL Register has been active [17], with an incidence of 10 cases per 100,000 inhabitants per year.

These figures on the incidence of ISSNHL in about 10–20 cases per 100,000 inhabitants per year would mean that there are about 4000–8000 new cases of ISSNHL each year in Spain, that is, about 20–80 cases each year for a level II hospital, which serves an average population of about 250,000 inhabitants. However, this incidence is increasing as our knowledge and concern of this disease grow, although there are notable geographical differences.

National ISSNHL Register

In January 2021, with the support of the Audiology Commission of the Spanish Society of Otorhinolaryngology and Head & Neck Surgery, the National ISSNHL Register was formally launched, a project in which more than 100 hospitals from all over Spain are taking part. As of 30 June 2023, 689 cases had been collected in 30 months for future analysis on the incidence rate in Spain. We have found an incidence of 25–35 cases per 100,000 per year in certain geographical areas in Spain that have been prospectively monitored (unpublished data).

In this Spanish ISSNHL Register, the mean age was 54.43 years, with a similar distribution by sex. In 35.37% of cases, ISSNHL was presented with associated tinnitus. The mean time to initiation of treatment was 15.31 days. Regarding complementary tests, magnetic resonance imaging (MRI) was requested in 95% of cases, although in 93% of cases no etiological diagnosis was concluded.

Risk Factors for Developing ISSNHL

The incidence of ISSNHL varies by age, sex, month of the year and season. Regarding age, the incidence gradually increases up to the age of 50 (Fig. 2), when its incidence skyrockets up to the age of 70, when it begins to fall. In relation to sex, there are no significant differences [18].

Meanwhile, there seems to be a direct relationship of ISSNHL cases with the coldest months of the year, which would be justified by the increase in respiratory infections during these periods. Thus, in the paper by the South Korean researcher Kim et al. [12], an annual incidence of 17.76/100,000 inhabitants per year was observed. The incidence per month was 1.48/100,000 inhabitants (standard deviation 0.39). The month with the lowest incidence was January (1.28/100,000). The peak month was October (1.65/100,000), which, due to South Korea's geographical location, is the coldest of the year and also when more respiratory infections are

Fig. 2 Higher incidence of ISSNHL between 60 and 80 years of age. Modified from Heuschkel et al. [18]

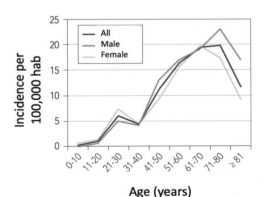

recorded. However, other studies have not been able to confirm a clear seasonality in the incidence of ISSNHL [19–25].

Association of ISSNHL with Other Conditions

Numerous studies have been published in recent years, especially from large databases in China, South Korea and Taiwan, which show a higher incidence of ISSNHL (odds ratio [OR] with significant confidence interval) in certain groups of patients with previous or concomitant conditions. The actual clinical significance of these associations should therefore be assessed (Table 2) [8].

Table 2 Association of ISSNHL with other clinical entities

Anxiety (Chung SD et al. 2015: OR 1.49)
Asthma (Choi HG et al. 2022: HR 1.23)
Rheumatoid arthritis (Lee SY et al. 2019: HR 1.4)
Nasopharyngeal carcinoma (Lin C et al. 2014: OR 6.53)
Tension headache (Hsiao et al. 2015: OR 1.86)
Depression (Kim JY et al. 2018: HR 1.66)
Post-ISSNHL erectile dysfunction (Hsu et al. 2013: HR 1.94)
Periodontal disease (Wu CS et al. 2013: OR 1.44))
Chronic kidney disease (Lin C et al. 2013: HR 1.46)
Iron deficiency (Chung SD et al. 2014: OR 1.34)
Hepatitis (Chen HC et al. 2017: OR 5.7)
Hypercholesterolaemia (Chang SL et al. 2014: OR 1.62; Simões et al. 2022: OR 2.09)
Previous SHL of other causes, not ISSNHL or Ménière's disease (Koo et al. 2015: OR 6.05)
Pre-ISSNHL myocardial infarction (Keller et al. 2013: OR 1.5)
Post-ISSNHL myocardial infarction (Crowson et al. 2017; Kim SY et al. 2018; Lin C et al. 2013): no higher incidence than in the general population
Human immunodeficiency virus (HIV) infection (Lin C et al. 2013: HR 2.1)
Human papillomavirus (HPV) infection (Chen TYT et al. 2022; HR 1.37)
Post-ISSNHL insomnia (Yeo CD et al. 2022; HR 1.4)
Vertebrobasilar insufficiency (Hsu et al. 2016: OR 1.76)
Pre-ISSNHL stroke (Kuo et al. 2016: OR 1.71)
Post-ISSNHL stroke (Khosravipour and Rajati meta-analysis 2021: HR 1.31):   – Chang CF et al. (2013): no higher incidence than in the general population (0.6% per year)   – Kim JY et al. (2018): no higher incidence than in the general population (HR 2.02)   – Oussoren et al. (2023): higher risk of stroke compared to controls (HR 1.22–4.08)
Gallstone (Chiu et al. 2015: OR 1.42)
Systemic lupus erythematosus (Lin C et al. 2013: HR 2.2)
Post-ISSNHL central retinal vein occlusion (Kim JY et al. 2022; HR 1.13)
Osteoporosis (Kim SY et al. 2018: HR 1.56)
Chronic otitis media (Yen YC et al. 2015: HR 3.02).
Migraine (Arslan et al. 2017; Chu et al. 2013: HR 1.8)
Mitral valve prolapse (Cheng YF et al. 2018: OR 1.69)

Table 2 (continued)

Psoriasis (Yen YC et al. 2015: HR 1.51; Ger et al. 2023; OR 1.45)
Metabolic syndrome (Chien et al. 2015: OR 3.54; Jung et al. 2018; Park JS et al. 2022; OR 4.3)
Chronic sinusitis (Hung et al. 2016: OR 1.36)
Previous use of statins (Chung SD et al. 2015: OR 1.36)

ISSNHL idiopathic sudden sensorineural hearing loss, *HR* hazard rate, *OR* odds ratio

Conclusions

Sudden sensorineural hearing loss, whether partial or total, unilateral or bilateral, is a condition which occurs suddenly and without a clear trigger. When the cause is not observed, it is defined as idiopathic SSNHL (ISSNHL).

We should take note of the increased incidence of ISSNHL because it will become more and more frequent both in medical appointments and in ENT emergencies. A better identification of patients with ISSNHL will be beneficial for better management of this condition [26].

This increase seems to be due to the ageing of the population, and therefore to the increase in accompanied risk factors, society's awareness of the condition and the improvement of patient access to the healthcare system.

Most cases of ISSNHL occur between the ages of 50 and 70, with it being rarer outside this range. Cold months and seasons can be triggers for ISSNHL episodes, depending on the geographical location. However, in general it has not been possible to demonstrate a clear seasonality in the incidence of ISSNHL.

References

1. Plaza G, Durio E, Herráiz C, Asociación Madrileña de ORL, et al. Consenso sobre el diagnóstico y tratamiento de la sordera súbita. Acta Otorrinolaringol Esp. 2011;62:144–57.
2. Herrera M, García Berrocal JR, García Arumí A, et al. Update on consensus on diagnosis and treatment of idiopathic sudden sensorineural hearing loss. Acta Otorrinolaringol Esp (Engl Ed). 2019;70:290–300.
3. Chandrasekhar SS, Tsai Do BS, Schwartz SR, et al. Clinical practice guideline: sudden hearing loss (update). Otolaryngol Head Neck Surg. 2019;161(Suppl. 1):S1–S45.
4. Fetterman BL, Luxford WM, Saunders JE. Sudden bilateral sensorineural hearing loss. Laryngoscope. 1996;106:1347–50.
5. Rauch SD. Clinical practice. Idiopathic sudden sensorineural hearing loss. N Engl J Med. 2008;359:833–40.
6. Stachler RJ, Chandrasekhar SS, Archer SM, American Academy of Otolaryngology-Head and Neck Surgery, et al. Clinical practice guideline: sudden hearing loss. Otolaryngol Head Neck Surg. 2012;146(Suppl. 3):S1–35.
7. De Kleyn A. Sudden complete or partial loss of function of the octavus system in apparently normal persons. Acta Otol. 1944;32:407–29.
8. Plaza G. Sordera súbita: diagnóstico y tratamiento. Madrid: Ergon; 2018.

9. Byl F. Thirty-two cases of sudden profound hearing loss occurring in 1973: incidence and prognostic findings. Trans Sect Otolaryngol Am Acad Ophthalmol Otolaryngol. 1975;80:298–305.

10. Byl FM. Sudden hearing loss: eight years' experience and suggested prognosis table. Laryngoscope. 1984;94:647–61.

11. Nakashima T, Tanabe T, Yanagita N, et al. Risk factors for sudden deafness: a case-control study. Auris Nasus Larynx. 1997;24:265–70.

12. Kim SH, Kim SJ, Im H, et al. A trend in sudden sensorineural hearing loss: data from a population-based study. Audiol Neurootol. 2017;22:311–6.

13. Alexander TH, Harris JP. Incidence of sudden sensorineural hearing loss. Otol Neurotol. 2013;34:1586–9.

14. Nomura Y. Diagnostic criteria for sudden deafness, mumps deafness and perilymphatic fistula. Acta Otolaryngol (Stockh). 1988;105(Suppl. 456):7–8.

15. Kitaoku Y, Tanaka M, Miyahara H, et al. Epidemiological survey of sudden deafness in Nara Prefecture in Japan. Pract Otorhinolaryngol. 1997;90:289–95.

16. Klemm E, Deutscher A, Mösges R. A present investigation of the epidemiology in idiopathic sudden sensorineural hearing loss. Laryngorhinootologie. 2009;88:524–7.

17. Nosrati-Zarenoe R, Arlinger S, Hultcrantz E. Idiopathic sudden sensorineural hearing loss: results drawn from the Swedish national database. Acta Otolaryngol. 2007;127:1168–75.

18. Heuschkel A, Geißler K, Boeger D, et al. Inpatient treatment of patients with idiopathic sudden sensorineural hearing loss: a population-based healthcare research study. Eur Arch Otorrinolaringol. 2018;275:699–707.

19. Danielides V, Nousia CS, Bartzokas A, et al. Weather conditions and sudden sensorineural hearing loss. BMC Ear Nose Throat Disord. 2002;2:2.

20. Lin HC, Lee HC, Chao PZ, Wu CS. The effects of weather on the incidence of sudden sensorineural hearing loss: a 5-year population-based study. Audiol Neurootol. 2006;11:165–71.

21. Jourdy DN, Donatelli LA, Victor JD, et al. Assessment of variation throughout the year in the incidence of idiopathic sudden sensorineural hearing loss. Otol Neurotol. 2010;31:53–7.

22. Seo JH, Jeon EJ, Park YS, et al. Meteorological conditions related to the onset of idiopathic sudden sensorineural hearing loss. Yonsei Med J. 2014;55:1678–82.

23. Zhang J, Ji S, Ma X, et al. Association between meteorological factors and audiogram configurations in patients with sudden sensorineural hearing loss: a cross-sectional study. BMJ Open. 2021;11:e045768.

24. Tal O, Ibrahim N, Ronen O. Assessment of seasonal pattern of idiopathic sudden sensorineural hearing loss—a retrospective cross-sectional study. J Laryngol Otol. 2023;137:515–9.

25. Simani L, Oron Y, Shapira U, et al. Is idiopathic sudden sensorineural hearing loss seasonal? Otol Neurotol. 2022;43:1016–21.

26. Yoon CY, Kong TH, Lee J, et al. Epidemiology of idiopathic sudden sensorineural hearing loss in the era of big data. Eur Arch Otorrinolaringol. 2023;280:2181–90.

Aetiology of Sudden Sensorineural Hearing Loss: Autoimmune Hypothesis

José Ramón García Berrocal, Ana Sánchez Martínez, Almudena Trinidad Cabezas, Antonio Rodríguez Valiente, Nuria Arnáiz Canora, and David R. Lobo Duro

Concept

Acceptance of immune-mediated inner ear disease (IMIED) as its own clinical entity was first published in 1979 [1], based on the clinical profile and response to steroid and immunosuppressive drug treatment. In animal models, it has been possible to establish an implication of the theories usually accepted in the aetiopathogenesis of idiopathic sudden sensorineural hearing loss (ISSNHL): vascular, viral and autoimmune. As a result, the viral infection triggers not only an involvement of the cochlear microvascularisation but also a powerful immune response inside the inner ear with the result of a fibro-osseous matrix, responsible for irreversible damage to the auditory organ. These lesions have been described in various systemic autoimmune diseases, in which a viral infection can be the triggering event of this disease. However, the low profitability of serological studies to identify different viruses in sudden hearing loss discourages their inclusion in the study protocol of this entity [2, 3].

For years, it was thought that the inner ear was isolated from humoral and cellular immunity by the blood–labyrinth barrier. However, it was possible to

---

J. R. García Berrocal (✉) · A. Trinidad Cabezas
Ear, Nose and Throat Department, Hospital Universitario Puerto de Hierro, Majadahonda, Madrid, Spain

Universidad Autónoma de Madrid, Madrid, Spain

A. Sánchez Martínez · A. Rodríguez Valiente · N. Arnáiz Canora
Ear, Nose and Throat Department, Hospital Universitario Puerto de Hierro, Majadahonda, Madrid, Spain

D. R. Lobo Duro
Ear, Nose and Throat Department, Hospital Universitario Marqués de Valdecilla, Santander, Cantabria, Spain

Valdecilla Biomedical Research Institute, Santander, Cantabria, Spain

G. Plaza, J. R. García Berrocal (eds.), *Sudden Sensorineural Hearing Loss*,
https://doi.org/10.1007/978-3-031-61385-2_2

demonstrate the existence of a local immune response in the inner ear, presumably initiated and enhanced in the endolymphatic sac, with recruitment of immunocompetent cells from the bloodstream, coming from Waldeyer's lymphatic ring. The immunological theory is based on the fact that antigens of the inner ear react with certain circulating antibodies or immunocomplexes or with activated T cells, causing damage to this organ [4]. A large number of internal ear antigens have been proposed as targets of the immune system attack, such as type II collagen, beta-actin, cochlin, beta-tectorin, P0 protein and choline transporter-like protein 2, among others. Immunoglobulins against support cells (DEP-1/CD148) and against connexin 26 (gap-junction protein) have been described in Cogan's syndrome [5].

ISSNHL can be considered the result of abnormal activation of cellular stress pathways involving the nuclear factor κβ in supporting cells and in the fibrocytes of the spiral ligament, causing the production of proinflammatory cytokines, including TNF-alpha, which would cause a rupture of the inner ear homeostasis, as these cells participate in the transport of K+ [6]. TNF-alpha induces a pro-constrictive state in cochlear circulation, causing a decrease in blood flow and, ultimately, cochlear ischaemia.

Likewise, ISSNHL can be an initial manifestation of systemic autoimmune diseases, such as Cogan's syndrome, temporal arteritis, granulomatosis with polyangiitis, polyarteritis nodosa and systemic lupus erythematosus.

Major Histocompatibility Complex and ISSNHL

The association of the *human leukocyte antigen* (HLA) with particular diseases is one of the most intriguing aspects of the major histocompatibility complex (MHC), which is located in the short arm of chromosome 6 in humans. Proteins encoded by this region are involved in immune recognition and interaction between lymphoid cells and antigen-presenting cells (APCs). The class II haplotypes HLA-DQ2/DR3, HLADQ6/DR2 and HLA-DQ8/DR4 account for more than 90% of all autoimmune diseases.

The existence of bilateral ISSNHL has been associated with HLA A1-B8-DR3 [7], supporting the immunological theory in the pathogenesis of this pathological entity. According to Yeo et al. [8], the class II haplotypes HLA-DRB1 and -DQB1 are significantly higher in patients with ISSNHL. The haplotypes HLA-DQA1 01 and -DQB1 06 are also linked to a good prognosis. More studies are needed in order to establish a correlation between this pathological entity and HLA.

Clinical Diagnosis of Immune-Mediated Hearing Loss

Sudden sensorineural hearing loss with autoimmune origin does not have an initial clinical presentation that is distinguishable from ISSNHL. Only long-term monitoring, for at least 1 year, can identify it, along with laboratory tests and the possible coexistence of a systemic autoimmune disease, with it being possible for ISSNHL to be the first sign of said disease.

In all cases of IMIED, the main characteristic is the positive response to corticoids and the suspected immunological profile.

In the initial phases, IMIED may present sudden hearing loss, so asymmetric that it would be indistinguishable from ISSNHL (hours to days) or rapidly progressive bilateral hearing loss (weeks or months) (Table 1). As the disease progresses, episodes of sudden hearing loss may be repeated in the same ear or spontaneously triggered in the contralateral ear, or after attacks on the inner ear (neurinoma surgery, trauma).

Autoantibodies

The demonstration of autoantibodies against inner ear antigens would support the involvement of the immune system in the pathogenesis of ISSNHL. The initial determination of anti-nuclear antibodies, rheumatoid factor, anti-mitochondrial antibodies, anti-smooth muscle antibodies, anti-parietal cell antibodies, anti-sarcolemma antibodies, anti-laminin antibodies, anti-reticulin antibodies and anti-collagen-type antibodies showed such disparate results that it radically modified our study protocol, currently including only anti-nuclear antibodies, as they have a higher percentage of positivities in this group of patients [9].

Some authors have observed the presence of anti-endothelial antibodies in patients with ISSNHL [10]. An association between sudden hearing loss and antiphospholipid antibodies has been established in systemic lupus erythematosus [11]. Antiphospholipid antibodies can be induced by human viruses whose products can have a sequence homologous to the phospholipid-binding regions, which would trigger cross-reactivity. These antibodies have a pathogenic effect on platelets and vascular endothelial cells, activating the endothelial cells of cochlear blood flow or generating free radicals that would secondarily damage the endothelium, leading to the formation of local microthrombi and the subsequent acute ischaemia of the organ, which would cause sudden hearing loss. The dissolution of the thrombus and subsequent reperfusion of the labyrinth vessels hours or days after the thrombotic event could partially explain the clinical course of sudden hearing loss in this group of patients.

The elevation of antiphospholipid antibodies (33.3%), anti-HSP 70 (25.4%) and ANAs (25.4%) has been described in patients with ISSNHL with a higher prevalence than in the normal population [12], which supports the presumption that ISSNHL may have an immune-mediated origin.

Table 1 Clinical presentation of immune-mediated hearing loss

Repeated sudden hearing loss in the same ear: two or more episodes in a year
Single-sided sudden hearing loss after previous involvement in the contralateral (sudden hearing loss, eighth neuroma surgery, lightning injury, trauma)

Patients with ISSNHL who have undergone a western blot test to detect anti-cochlear antibodies in the 68–70 kDa positive band have a better prognosis of response to steroid treatment than those who have tested negative [13]. However, the low reactivity to heat shock protein 70 (HSP-70) shown in patients with ISSNHL [14] suggested that it should be terminated in the routine immunological study developed in our group.

A systematic analysis of literature [15] supports the increased performance of the immune panel described above, including only antinuclear antibodies.

Immunophenotyping of Peripheral Blood Lymphocytes

After conducting an analysis of T cells by flow cytometry, the most frequently detected alterations appear in the CD4+, CD8+ and CD4+/CD8+ populations [16], suggesting that a subset of patients with ISSNHL behaves as an immune deficiency. Our research shows a decrease in CD4+ (T helper lymphocytes), CD8+ (cytotoxic-suppressor T lymphocytes) and naïve T cells (CD4+ CD45RA+ and CD8+ CD45RA+) [16].

Patients with ISSNHL and positive response to steroid treatment showed a tendency to normalise such populations. However, the group with poor response showed an increase in CD4+ CD45RO+ memory T cells and low levels of CD8+ CD45RA+ -naïve cells. These differences may indicate the persistence of the antigen/s triggering the immune response, with a continued transformation of naïve CD4+ cells into memory cells despite treatment. In addition, the existence of a deficient population of cytotoxic naïve cells could suggest a priori a poor response to treatment as there is a deficiency of cytotoxic mechanisms.

These abnormalities are similar to those described in other autoimmune diseases, although the underlying causes of various autoimmune diseases may be different. Thus, the deficiency of naïve cells could be justified by the existence of autoantibodies against them; the conversion of naïve cells into memory cells as a result of the onset of the immune response; or the viral infection of these cells, which is difficult to demonstrate as there is a minimum percentage of seroconversions against the most frequent respiratory viruses or perhaps expresses the recruitment of these cells to the sites of focal inflammation, in this case the inner ear.

Magnetic Resonance Imaging (MRI)

Initially, the MRI study of sudden hearing loss sought to rule out the existence of a tumour of a cerebellopontine angle and/or internal auditory canal as approximately 14% of these neoplasms, mostly schwannomas of the vestibular nerve, may debut as sudden hearing loss.

However, in a patient suffering from atypical Cogan's syndrome who presented with sudden bilateral anacusis after upper airway catarrh, a hyperintensity of the membranous labyrinth on pre-contrast T1-weighted images was observed at 48 h compared to the vestibulocochlear nerve [17]. This finding represents a different contribution to the aetiopathogenic mechanism of IMIED and is compatible with the rupture of the blood–labyrinth barrier, possibly secondary to circulating immunocomplexes developed by cross-response with the virus responsible for the systemic presentation.

Recent studies have confirmed these high-intensity signals in the affected ear in pre-contrast and post-contrast 3D-FLAIR MRI, suggesting three different radiological patterns, correlated with mild bleeding, acute inflammation and presence or absence of rupture of the blood–labyrinth barrier or nerve barrier [18].

Hence the suggestion to perform an MRI in the first month after the ISSNHL triggering event, preferably in the first two weeks. A study with more patients could conclude that the findings of the MRI study would support the immune-mediated aetiology, with it even being a criterion in the diagnostic profile of this group of patients.

In cases of repeat ISSNHL, the existence of endolymphatic hydrops should be ruled out, which can be demonstrated by MRI with intratympanic gadolinium [19].

Diagnostic Criteria for Immune-Mediated Sudden Sensorineural Hearing Loss

The impact of early diagnosis and treatment on hearing recovery, coupled with the absence of sufficiently sensitive serologic testing, forces immunomodulatory therapy to be initiated without delay based on the clinical characteristics of the patient affected by immune-mediated ISSNHL.

On the basis of the immunological study, the profile of immune-mediated hearing loss was proposed and subsequently confirmed by extending the studies to a greater number of patients (Table 2) [20].

The fulfilment of three major criteria, or two major criteria plus two minor ones, would support the diagnosis of suspected immune-mediated involvement, considering that losses >90 dB are difficult to recover, regardless of their aetiology.

A recent review modified the initial profile, validating it when three criteria are met:

Table 2 Diagnostic criteria for immune-mediated sudden sensorineural hearing loss

Major criteria
1. Bilateral involvement
2. Presence of systemic autoimmune disease
3. High level of antinuclear antibodies (ANAs)
4. Reduced number of naïve T cells (CD4 + CD45 + RA) versus memory T cells (CD4 + CD45 + RO)
5. Hearing recovery rate above 80%
Minor criteria
1. Unilateral involvement
2. Young or middle-aged female patient
3. Positivity to heat shock protein 70 (HSP70)
4. Positive response to steroid treatment (<80% recovery)

- Clinical course: two or more episodes in a year and/or bilateral onset.
- Presence of antinuclear autoantibodies (ANAs) > 1/160.
- Altered T cell immunophenotyping.
- Response to corticosteroids (oral or intratympanic) in each episode (except in cases with profound hearing loss).
- Possible association with systemic autoimmune diseases.

The involvement of organs other than the inner ear after diagnosing IMIED would suggest the need for collaboration with other specialists (rheumatologists, internists) to address the treatment in a consensual and multidisciplinary way.

The use of PET, which has been shown to be useful in some systemic autoimmune diseases, means that IMIED can be classified as primary (when the only organ affected is the ear) and secondary (when other organs are also involved [21].

Research into the role of certain cytokines (IL-16, IL-17, etc.) will mean that their use in the diagnostic profile can be implemented.

Treatment of Immune-Mediated Sudden Sensorineural Hearing Loss

Corticoids are the gold standard in the treatment of immune-mediated SSNHL as they have an excellent effect unmatched by any other immunomodulatory drug. In addition, the positive response is one of the criteria used for the diagnosis of this pathological entity, in which spontaneous recovery is highly unlikely.

Since this form of presentation is shared with ISSNHL and only patient follow-up can lead to a diagnosis of IMIED, the initial treatment will be the same for both pathological entities.

Based on the last consensus document published in 2019 [22], the initial treatment would follow this pattern:

- If diagnosis has been possible within 30 days of symptom onset, treatment will be by.
  - Intratympanic corticosteroids at ENT outpatient appointments:
    A weekly dose of 0.9–1 ml of methylprednisolone 40 mg/ml or dexamethasone 8 mg/ml, for 3–4 weeks (after topical anaesthesia by injecting the drug with a 27 g lumbar puncture needle). In some patients, it is necessary to shorten the interval of injections depending on the duration of the hearing gain.
  - As a second option, oral corticosteroids in one of these regimens:
    Prednisone (Prednisone Alonga®, Dacortin®), 1 mg/kg bodyweight/day, descending every 5 days (e.g., in a patient weighing 80 kg: 80 mg × 5 days; 60 mg × 5 days; 40 mg × 5 days; 20 mg × 5 days; 10 mg × 5 days; 5 mg × 5 days).
    Methylprednisolone (Urbason®), 1 mg/kg bodyweight/day, descending every 5 days (e.g., in a patient weighing 80 kg: 80 mg × 5 days;

     60 mg × 5 days; 40 mg × 5 days; 20 mg × 5 days; 10 mg × 5 days; 5 mg × 5 days).

     Deflazacort (Dezacor®, Zamene®), in a similar descending pattern, 1.5 mg/kg bodyweight/day, descending every 5 days (e.g., in a patient weighing 80 kg: 120 mg × 5 days; 90 mg × 5 days; 60 mg × 5 days; 30 mg × 5 days; 15 mg × 5 days).

- In the case of severe SSNHL (>70 dB) in one ear or with associated intense vertigo, intravenous treatment with corticosteroids will be offered for 5 days, either at outpatients or by hospital admission, with a 500 mg dose of methylprednisolone per day with slow administration of saline solution in 30 min. Subsequently, the oral regimen described above would be reintroduced.

During treatment with systemic steroids, either oral or intravenous, gastroduodenal prophylaxis will be performed with proton pump inhibitors with omeprazole at a dose of 40 mg /day for 1 month.

In patients over 65 years of age, if the glucocorticoid treatment lasts more than 15 days, it will be necessary to combine vitamin D (800 IU/day) and calcium (800–1000 mg/day) as a preventive regimen of bone mass loss and osteoporosis, with the option of requesting a bone densitometry.

Informed consent is required for both intratympanic corticosteroids and intravenous mega-pulses.

Follow-Up

Once the treatment has been established, a check-up is carried out 1 week after the start of the treatment, including pure tone and speech audiometry exams, to assess tolerance to the treatment and its results. Pure tone and speech audiometry exams are performed at 15, 30 and 90 days after diagnosis, although to rule out autoimmune hearing loss or Ménière's disease it would be advisable to check patients up to 1 year after diagnosis, especially in hearing losses that affect low frequencies.

Once possible immune-mediated SSNHL has been diagnosed, the treatment regimen for subsequent hearing fluctuations may include

- Oral prednisone 1 mg/kg/day for 15 days:
  - Decrease of 10 mg/week until reaching 30 mg/day.
  - Decrease of 5 mg/2 weeks until reaching 10 mg/day.
  - Decrease of 2.5 mg/2 weeks until reaching 2.5 mg/day.
  - 2.5 mg/day every other day until stopped.
- Intratympanic methylprednisolone (40 mg/ml): 1 injection weekly, 4 weeks with re-assessment and another cycle based on results (hearing stabilisation or not).

Other Treatments

The incorporation of new biological drugs into systemic autoimmune diseases (methotrexate, anti-TNF, azathioprine, anti-IL1, etc.) [23–25] has provided an encouraging therapeutic strategy in patients with hearing fluctuations that make it impossible for them to stop systemic steroid treatment, associated or not with intratympanic treatment, whose adverse effects may limit their continuous administration.

The application of therapeutic strategies that more selectively and effectively modulate the immune system will create new perspectives in the treatment of this pathological entity.

References

1. McCabe BF. Autoimmune sensorineural hearing loss. Ann Otol Rhinol Laryngol. 1979;88:585–9.
2. García-Berrocal JR, Ramírez-Camacho R, Portero F, et al. Role of viral and mycoplasma pneumoniae infection in idiopathic sudden sensorineural hearing loss. Acta Otolaryngol. 2000;120:835–9.
3. García-Berrocal JR, Ramírez-Camacho R, González-García JA, et al. Does the serological study for viral infection in autoimmune inner ear disease make sense? ORL. 2008;70:16–20.
4. García-Berrocal JR, Ramírez-Camacho R. Sudden sensorineural hearing loss: supporting the immunologic theory. Ann Otol Rhinol Laryngol. 2002;111:989–97.
5. Lunardi C, Bason C, Leandri M, et al. Autoantibodies to inner ear and endothelial antigens in Cogan's syndrome. Lancet. 2002;360:915–21.
6. García-Berrocal JR, Ramírez-Camacho R, Millán I, et al. Sudden presentation of immune-mediated inner ear disease: characterization and acceptance of a cochleovestibular dysfunction. J Laryngol Otol. 2003;117:775–9.
7. Psillas G, Daniilidis M, Gerofotis Veros AK, et al. Sudden bilateral sensorineural hearing loss associated with HLA A1-B8-DR3 Haplotype. Case Rep Otolaryngol. 2013;2013:590157.
8. Yeo SW, Chang K-H, Suh B-D, et al. Distribution of HLA-A, -B and -DRB1 alleles in patients with sudden sensorineural hearing loss. Acta Otolaryngol. 2000;120:710–5.
9. García-Berrocal JR, Trinidad A, Ramírez-Camacho R, et al. Immunologic work-up study for inner ear disorders: looking for a rational strategy. Acta Otolaryngol. 2005;125:814–8.
10. Ottaviani F, Cadoni G, Marinelli M, et al. Anti-endothelial autoantibodies in patients with sudden hearing loss. Laryngoscope. 1999;109:1084–7.
11. Naarendorp M, Spiera H. Sudden sensorineural hearing loss in patients with systemic lupus erythematosus or lupus-like syndromes and antiphospholipid antibodies. J Rheumatol. 1998;25:589–92.
12. Gross M, Eliashar R, Ben-Yaakov A, et al. Prevalence and clinical significance of anticardiolipin, Anti-2 -Glycoprotein-1, and anti-heat shock protein-70 autoantibodies in sudden sensorineural hearing loss. Audiol Neurotol. 2008;13:231–8.
13. García Callejo FJ, Velert Vila M, Laporta P, et al. Titulación de anticuerpos anticocleares mediante Western-Blot y grado de recuperación auditiva tras corticoterapia en pacientes con sordera súbita. Acta Otorrinolaringol Esp. 2004;55:463–9.
14. García Berrocal JR, Ramírez-Camacho R, Arellano B, et al. Validity of the Western blot immunoassay for heat shock protein 70 in associated and isolated immuno-related inner ear disease. Laryngoscope. 2002;112:304–9.
15. Lobo D, García López F, García-Berrocal JR, et al. Diagnostic tests for immunomediated hearing loss. J Laryngol Otol. 2008;122:564–73.

16. García-Berrocal JR, Vargas JA, Ramírez-Camacho R, et al. Deficiency of naive T cells in patients with sudden deafness. Arch Otolaryngol Head Neck Surg. 1997;123:712–7.
17. García-Berrocal JR, Vargas JA, Vaquero M, et al. Cogan's syndrome: an oculo-audiovestibular disease. Postgrad Med J. 1999;75:262–4.
18. Berrettini S, Seccia V, Fortunato S, et al. Analysis of the 3-dimensional fluid-attenuated inversion-recovery (3D-FLAIR) sequence in idiopathic sudden sensorineural hearing loss. JAMA Otolaryngol-Head Neck Surg. 2013;139:455–64.
19. Lobo D, Tuñón M, Villareal I, et al. Intratympanic gadolinium MRI can support the role of endolymphatic hydrops in immune-mediated inner ear disease. J Laryngol Otol. 2018;132:554–9.
20. García-Berrocal JR, Ramírez-Camacho R, Vargas JA, et al. Does the serological testing really play a role in the diagnosis of immune-mediated sensorineural hearing loss? Acta Otolaryngol. 2002;122:243–8.
21. Mucientes Rasilla J, Ann Field C, Ortiz Evan L, et al. ¿Puede la tomografía por emisión de positrones ayudar en la caracterización de la enfermedad inmunomediada del oído interno? Rev Esp Med Nucl Imagen Mol. 2018;37:290–5.
22. Herrera M, García Berrocal JR, García Arumí A, et al. Update on consensus on diagnosis and treatment of idiopathic sudden sensorineural hearing loss. Acta Otorrinolaringol Esp. 2019;70:290–300.
23. García-Berrocal JR, Ibáñez A, Rodríguez A, et al. Alternatives to systemic steroid therapy for refractory immune-mediated inner ear disease: a physiopathologic approach. Eur Arch Otorrinolaringol. 2006;263:977–82.
24. Lobo D, García-Berrocal JR, Trinidad A, et al. Revisión de las terapias biológicas en la enfermedad inmunomediada del oído interno. Acta Otorrinolaringol Esp. 2013;64:223–9.
25. Mata Castro N, Gavilanes Plasencia J, Ramírez Camacho R, et al. La azatioprina reduce el riesgo de recaída audiométrica en hipoacusia inmunomediada. Acta Otorrinolaringol Esp. 2018;69:260–7.

Aetiology of Sudden Sensorineural Hearing Loss: Vascular, Viral or due to Perilymphatic Fistula

Mayte Herrera and Guillermo Plaza

Introduction

The causes of sudden sensorineural hearing loss (SSNHL) are highly varied and in many cases multifactorial. Several possible aetiological theories have therefore been proposed, sometimes the result of speculation or of specific findings (Table 1) [1–7]. In most cases of SSNHL, there is no obvious cause, and then the disease is usually known as idiopathic sudden sensorineural hearing loss (ISSNHL) [6–8].

A historical review of the sequential evolution of the aetiopathogenic theories of ISSNHL is summarised in Fig. 1. Most likely, cochlear oxidative stress is the common link between such disparate causes as it affects all of them [9–13].

Following a systematic review of literature based on more than 30 articles, Chau et al. [8] concluded that the most common aetiologies of SSNHL are idiopathic (71%), infectious (12.8%), due to ear diseases (4.7%), trauma (4.2%), vascular or haematological diseases (2.8%), neoplasms (2.3%) and other causes (2.2%).

M. Herrera (✉)
Ear, Nose and Throat Department, Hospital Universitario de Fuenlabrada, Madrid, Spain

Ear, Nose and Throat Department, Hospital Universitario Sanitas La Zarzuela, Madrid, Spain

G. Plaza
Ear, Nose and Throat Department, Hospital Universitario de Fuenlabrada, Madrid, Spain

Ear, Nose and Throat Department, Hospital Universitario Sanitas La Zarzuela, Madrid, Spain

Universidad Rey Juan Carlos, Madrid, Spain

G. Plaza, J. R. García Berrocal (eds.), *Sudden Sensorineural Hearing Loss*, https://doi.org/10.1007/978-3-031-61385-2_3

Table 1 Causes of sudden sensorineural hearing loss

Infection	Trauma	Neoplasia	Autoimmune disorder
Epidemic meningitis Encephalitis Herpes virus (simplex, zoster, chickenpox, cytomegalovirus) Parotitis Measles HIV Lyme disease Rubella SARS-CoV-2 (COVID-19) Syphilis Toxoplasmosis	Barotrauma Perilymphatic fistula Exposure to intense noise Inner ear decompression Fracture of temporal bone Ear surgery (stapedectomy)	Tumours of the pontocerebellar angle (vestibular schwannoma) Leukaemia Myeloma	Granulomatosis with polyangiitis Rheumatoid arthritis Gougerout–Sjögren syndrome Polyarteritis nodosa Relapsing polychondritis Lupus erythematosus Ulcerative colitis Cogan's syndrome Antiphospholipid syndrome Sarcoidosis Autoimmune inner ear disease
Toxic	**Vascular**	**Neurological**	**Metabolic**
Aminoglycoside antibiotics Loop diuretics NSAIDs Salicylate Platinum-derived chemotherapies General anaesthesia	Vascular diseases/ altered microvascularisation Mitochondrial diseases (with vascular disorder) Vertebrobasilar insufficiency Erythrocyte deformity Sickle cell anaemia Cardiopulmonary bypass	Multiple sclerosis Focal pontine ischaemia Migraine	Hyperlipidaemia Thyrotoxicosis Diabetes

Fig. 1 Historical evolution of the aetiopathogenic theories of ISSNHL

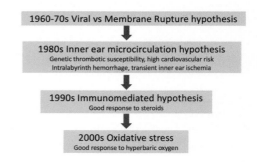

Vascular Aetiology

For many years, the most accepted theory to justify most cases of ISSNHL was the vascular hypothesis. The abrupt clinical picture that defines ISSNHL, the terminal blood supply of the inner ear, where the lack of distal anastomoses is evident [9, 11] (Fig. 2), the presence of accompanying otological symptoms, such as vertigo and instability with or without tinnitus, and the fact that in many patients it occurs during the early hours of the morning, suggest the existence of a vascular event as a cause [14].

In fact, up to three theoretical mechanisms have been described as causing vascular damage to the inner ear. In all of them, cochlear damage and dysfunction secondary to hypoxia would inevitably lead to ISSNHL [9]:

1. Permanent and total occlusion of arterial supply to the cochlea. This would cause necrosis of the labyrinth membranes, followed by fibrosis and ossification.
2. Total but temporary occlusion of the arterial vessels of the cochlea due to transient ischaemic phenomena.
3. Existence of low blood flow with consequent insufficient oxygenation for the metabolic requirements of the cochlea. This can happen in states of hyperviscosity such as hypergammaglobulinaemia, thrombocytosis, leukaemia or in states of hypercoagulability [15, 16].

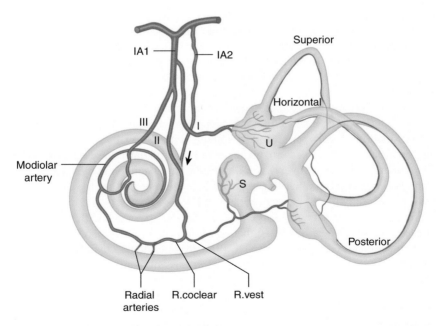

Fig. 2 Cochlear blood supply. (Taken from Hultcrantz [11]) IA1 = main internal auditory artery; I = anterior vestibular artery; II = cochleovestibular artery; III = cochlear artery; IA2 = accessory internal auditory artery (present in 50% of cases, and anastomosing with branch II of IA1)

However, the vascular theory for ischaemia as a cause of SSNHL presents several doubts [17]:

1. There is a discrepancy in the anatomopathological findings in the different studies between animals and humans.
2. The very nature of vascular theory contradicts the high number of cases with spontaneous recovery as most vascular events are more likely to be irreversible.
3. In experimental studies, cochlear microphonic and action potentials are affected with only 30 s of anoxia, while pathophysiologically it has been proved that changes in the inner ear occur over several hours and do not recover if the ischaemia lasts for longer than 72 h.
4. The high incidence in middle-aged patients contradicts the existence of cardiovascular risk factors, more common in elderly patients.
5. Finally, the involvement of more frequent high frequencies contradicts the terminal vascularisation of the cochlea, which is worse in the apical region.

On the other hand, from a clinical point of view, some cases of ISSNHL are clearly related to previous or concomitant vascular events. Thus, for example, ISSNHL has been linked to the existence of basilar and vertebral artery thrombosis associated with facial paralysis or pontine infarctions in which the only symptom is ISSNHL, sometimes bilateral [9].

Lin et al. [18] presented in 2012 a meta-analysis on risk factors and ISSNHL, collecting a total of 22 articles with sufficient quality. They confirmed that cardiovascular risk factors are associated with an increased risk of ISSNHL. Thus, in large population-based studies in Asian countries [19], patients who have had a stroke are more likely to have ISSNHL afterwards, with an OR of 1.71. Likewise, the probability of having a stroke increases after suffering ISSNHL [20], with an OR of 2.02.

Recently, Simões et al. [21] presented a meta-analysis including 19 case–control studies and 2 cohorts, determining a higher prevalence of hypercholesterolaemia, diabetes mellitus and hypertension in patients with ISSNHL, with an increase in triglycerides and total cholesterol being the factors with the highest risk for ISSNHL (OR 1.54 and 2.09, respectively). Similar results have been found by Saba et al. [22] in another meta-analysis, but Lenkeit et al. [23] did not find such association in a case–control study in 223 patients with ISSNHL.

There have also been numerous cases of ISSNHL associated with specific medical events in which it is suspected that there may be a microembolism or an ischaemic phenomenon that causes SSNHL [9]: cardiopulmonary bypass, possibly due to microembolisms during it; other surgical interventions in which there may be a risk of remote cochlear ischaemia; dental interventions; and anaesthetic interventions, especially epidural and haemodialysis [24].

In all these cases, the causal relationship between the vascular event and the development of ISSNHL is evident, perhaps due to hypotension and ischaemia, whether or not related to the use of nitrous oxide in anaesthesia, which may or may not be reversible when the event is resolved [25].

As proof of the current validity of vascular aetiology as a cause of ISSNHL, the use of hyperbaric oxygen therapy (HBOT) has been established and accepted. Several studies, including systematic reviews and meta-analyses, have shown that HBOT, as a combination treatment with corticosteroid therapy, is superior to isolated corticosteroid therapy, both as an initial and a salvage option [26–29]. Therefore, current consensus recommends HBOT [3, 5].

Infectious Aetiology

Viral Infection

Viral theory was for many years one of the most credible and accepted cause of ISSNHL. In 1977, Mattox and Simmons [30] described the presence of a viral history 1 month before the start of SSNHL in 28% of cases. Currently, although the association has not been definitively demonstrated, viral cochleitis is for many authors the justification for most cases of ISSNHL.

For other authors, however, it is more of a circumstantial association, given that there is a moderate incidence of intercurrent upper-airway catarrhal processes in patients with ISSNHL, which does not differ much from that in other patients who visit an otolaryngologist for other conditions. Moreover, the patient's immunity conditions, and not the viral presence itself, may well determine the occurrence of ISSNHL [9].

Many authors have attempted to find higher seroconversion rates in patients with ISSNHL compared with controls for numerous viruses, such as influenza B, enterovirus and herpes simplex virus (HSV) type I (Table 2). In 1983, Wilson et al. [31] reviewed 122 patients over a 3-year period and found a seroconversion of 40% compared to controls and a higher prevalence in the spring.

Table 2 Viral relation to ISSNH[L]

Studies	%	Association with SSNHL
Maasab et al. (1973)	62	Adenovirus
Jaffe (1978)	61.7	Adenovirus
Mercke et al. (1980)	6	Adenovirus
Veltri et al. (1981)	65	Influenza B, measles
Wilson et al. (1983)	63	Parotitis, measles, VZV, CMV, influenza B
Schulz et al. (1998)	100	HSV-1
Pitkaranta et al. (1998)	0	No
Gagnebin et al. (2000)	0	No
García-Berrocal et al. (2000)	12.5	No
Mishra et al. (2005)	18.75	No
López et al. (2011)	60	Respiratory syncytial virus
Scalia et al. (2013)	40	igA HSV-1
Park et al. (2017)	No	HSV-1 reactivation
Lan et al. (2023)	10.3	Epstein–Barr virus (real-time PCR)

More recently, Gross et al. [32] could not find any cases of seroconversion associated with ISSNHL. In Kathmandu, Mishra et al. [33] analysed 32 cases of ISSNHL and 10 controls, looking for seroconversion due to various viruses. In total, 22% of patients demonstrated some seropositivity for mumps (12%) and herpes zoster (10%).

However, the association to viruses is much less commonly cited in the ISSNHL series in recent years [34, 35]·López et al. [36] reviewed a case series of ISSNHL in Chile, observing that in 60% of cases there were nasopharyngeal cultures positive for viruses, including respiratory syncytial virus and herpesvirus. Scalia et al. [37] reported that IgA to HSV was very common in ISSNHL, while Park et al. [38] have shown that HSV reactivation was not associated to ISSNHL. Recently, Lan et al. [39] have also showed Epstein–Barr virus to be related to ISSNHL [36]·

The proposed mechanisms for inner ear viral lesion in ISSNHL include direct viral invasion, reactivation of latent viruses in the spiral ganglion (especially the herpes virus) and immune-mediated mechanisms. Viral particles can only be discovered in postmortem studies, so today this theory remains unproven in many cases. Even so, there are anatomopathological studies that support this theory more than the vascular theory, given that the findings in the inner ear are more compatible with a viral lesion [9, 34].

Initially proposed by Hughes et al. [40], the use of antivirals has been systematically reviewed by Cochrane [41], including a meta-analysis of four published randomised clinical trials of 257 ISSNHL cases. Its conclusions were that the efficacy of antivirals in ISSNHL has not been demonstrated, so current consensus does not recommend them [3, 5].

Other Infectious Agents

- Mycoplasma pneumoniae: Its low incidence does not warrant serological screening [42].
- Lyme disease: positive Serological titres for *Borrelia burgdorferi*, the causative agent of this disease, may be elevated by up to 20% in patients with ISSNHL in endemic areas. However, there were no significant differences between clinical findings and the possibility of recovery in patients with positive or negative serological titres. Therefore, it is not recommended to include its routine study in patients with SSNHL, except in endemic areas [43, 44].
- Syphilis: Its low incidence does not warrant a general serological screening, but it may be interesting in certain patients with suspected clinical history or symptoms [45, 46].

ISSNHL and COVID-19

Regarding ISSNHL in the context of SARS-CoV-2 (COVID-19) infection, there have been numerous reports of isolated cases of ISSNHL, although the aetiopathogenesis of damage to the inner ear that this virus may cause is unknown [47–51]. Fancello et al. [52] conducted a review from March 2020 to April 2021 and found that sensorineural hearing loss is the most frequent ENT symptom along with tinnitus and vertigo. However, several studies in the United States, the Netherlands and Israel failed to demonstrate a higher frequency of ISSNHL during the pandemic [53–55]. In fact, there was a decrease in cases during the first wave of the pandemic, which could be partly justified by the lack of emergency assistance during this period [56, 57]. Likewise, there was also less incidence during the rest of the pandemic, possibly due to the use of facemasks and social distancing [57].

Regarding vaccination against SARS-CoV-2, isolated cases were also reported, but several reviews failed to confirm a clear relationship between vaccination and ISSNHL [58–64]. A recent meta-analysis included a total of 630 patients with a mean age of 57.3. Of the patients, 328 out of 609 vaccinated patients took the Pfizer-BioNTech BNT162b2 vaccine, while 242 (40%) took the Moderna COVID-19 vaccine. The mean time from vaccination to hearing impairment was 6.2 days, ranging from a few hours to 1 month after the last dose. The results found a significant difference between vaccine types in terms of incidence and prognosis of the condition, while they showed that the number of doses prior to the onset had no significance. However, the COVID-19 vaccine has been demonstrated to be safe and effective in preventing illness, and the benefits of vaccination are significant compared to any potential risks [65].

Traumatic Aetiology: Disruption of Membranes

It is evident that barotrauma can cause deafness and that a perilymphatic fistula can cause ISSNHL. Therefore, even in the absence of known barotrauma, the theory of disruption of the round window membrane as a cause of ISSNHL emerged 50 years ago. Thus, Goodhill recognised the development of a perilymphatic fistula as a possible origin of SSNHL and proposed the main mechanisms in its formation [66].

The round window is the only soft-tissue barrier between the inner and middle ear. It is semi-permeable and has a thickness of approximately 60–70 μm. It is presumed that the rupture of this window conditions the existence of perilymph in the middle ear. This could be detected by CT as the accumulation of fluid around the niche of the window [67].

Three criteria are described in the literature to confirm the existence of a rupture of the round window during the surgical exploration of the middle ear: direct observation of a fistula with perilymphatic exit, direct vision of a rupture of the round window or a failure in ear windows game. However, in many of the articles describing the sealing of such fistula, none of the three criteria was found during surgery [9].

Even so, there is a growing interest in the use of exploratory tympanotomy with sealing of the round window, whether or not a perilymphatic fistula is seen, as salvage treatment when the usual treatment has not been effective. This treatment is especially recommended in severe or profound hearing loss alongside vertigo and in patients under 65 years of age [68]. However, in the case of invasive treatment, the possible spontaneous recovery of ISSNHL makes it prudent to wait for a few days before indicating exploratory tympanotomy, but still within the first 5–10 days [68–73].

Thomas et al. [72] reviewed 136 cases of ISSNHL treated by exploratory tympanotomy, obtaining hearing improvement in 77% of cases, and observing that a history of pressure change entails a factor of good prognosis (OR 4.6). Heilen et al. [73] published a recent literature review including eight studies with more than 300 cases in total and 90 cases of their own, in which fistula is only observed in an average of 13.6% of exploratory tympanotomies, without significant hearing improvement being observed, whether there is a fistula present or not.

In the current clinical guide for ISSNHL in Germany [12], after 3 days with intravenous treatment with prednisolone at initial doses of 250 mg/day (range 100–500 mg/day), exploratory tympanotomy is recommended if severe hearing loss persists (>80 dB), while intratympanic salvage with steroids should be considered when the threshold is between 40 and 80 dB (Fig. 3). In contrast, current consensus in the United States, Spain and China does not recommend exploratory tympanotomy as a treatment for ISSNHL (Table 3) [3, 5, 74].

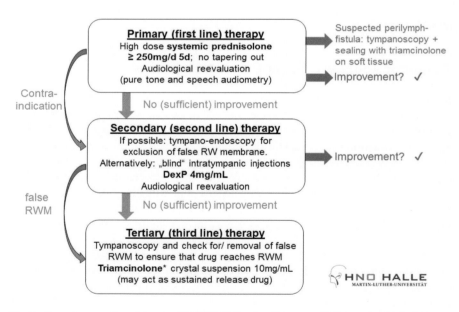

Fig. 3 Staged approach to therapy of ISSNHL following German guidelines using high-dose systemic steroids followed by exploratory tympanotomy. *RWM* round window membrane. (Taken from Plontke SK. Diagnostics and therapy of sudden hearing loss. GMS Curr Top Otorhinolaryngol Head Neck Surg. 2017; 16: 1–21 (http://creativecommons.org/licenses/by/4.0/))

Table 3 Comparison of key information in current SSNHL guidelines

	China	USA	Germany	Spain
Agency	CMA	AAOHNS	AWMF	SEORL
Year of publication	2015	2019	2014	2019
Audiological criteria	A decrease ≥20 dB affecting at least 2 consecutive frequencies	A decrease ≥30 dB affecting at least 3 consecutive frequencies	Not specified	A decrease ≥30 dB affecting at least 3 consecutive frequencies
Classification	Classified into four types by frequency and severity of hearing loss	Not specified	Classified into five types by frequency and severity of hearing loss	Classified into five types by frequency and severity of hearing loss
Supporting tests	Necessary: otoscopy, tuning fork test/pure tone audiometry Nystagmus examination (when accompanied by vertigo) As required: OAE/ABR/ECochG, imaging examination, laboratory testing	Recommendation: history and physical examination, pure tone and speech audiometry, retrocochlear pathology (MRI/ABR) Strong recommendation against: CT of the head, laboratory tests	Necessary: history, otoscopy, tuning fork test/pure tone and speech audiometry, Nystagmus examination As required: OAE/Stapedius reflex, cervical spine, Imaging examination, laboratory testing, ASSR, etc.	Necessary: History, Otoscopy, Tuning fork test/Pure tone and Speech Audiometry, Nystagmus examination Necessary: As required: Imaging examination, Laboratory testing
Steroid therapy	Systemic application: prednisone at 1 mg/kg/d for 3–5 days	Systemic application: prednisone at 1 mg/kg/d for 7–14 days, then taper over	Systemic application: prednisolone at 250 mg/d for 3 days	Systemic application: prednisone at 1 mg/kg/d for 7–14 days, then taper over
	Local application: ITS/PAS as salvage treatment	Local application: ITS as initial or salvage treatment	Local application: ITS as salvage treatment	Local application: ITS as initial or salvage treatment

(continued)

Table 3 (continued)

	China	USA	Germany	Spain
Combination therapy	Recommendation: vasodilators, hemorheology	Optional: hyperbaric oxygen therapy	Optional: Vasodilators, Hemor. and Exploratory tympanotomy	Optional: Hyperbaric oxygen therapy
	Against: hyperbaric oxygen therapy	Against: other pharmacologic therapy	Not specified: Hyperbaric oxygen therapy	
			Against: Hydroxyethyl starch	

CMA Chinese Medical Association, *AAOHNS* American Academy of Otolaryngology-Head and Neck Surgery, *AWMF* Arbeitsgemeinschaft Wissenschaftlich Medizinischer Fachgesellschaften (Association of Scientific Medical Societies in Germany), *OAE* otoacoustic emission; *ECochG* electrocochleogram, *SEORL* Sociedad Española de Otorrinolaringología (Spanish ENT Society), *ITS* intratympanic steroids, *PAS* postauricular steroids
Viral relation to ISSNHL

Conclusions

SSNHL is a multifactorial disease. Differential diagnosis should rule out specific causes of SSNHL, which require a specific treatment and may have a better prognosis [75].

When the cause is not found, SSNHL is idiopathic (ISSNHL). Beyond the autoimmune aetiology of ISSNHL, some cases have a clearly vascular, ischaemic or thrombotic origin [76]. Others are related to infections, most often viral. Other patients have ISSNHL in relation to a perilymphatic fistula.

In the differential diagnosis of ISSNHL, the ENT specialist should consider the different possible aetiologies, carefully assessing clinical history and findings in complementary tests, in order to rule out the causes that can be treated specifically, such as vascular or labyrinthine fistula.

References

1. Rauch SD. Clinical practice. Idiopathic sudden sensorineural hearing loss. N Engl J Med. 2008;359:833–40.
2. Plaza G, Durio E, Herráiz C, Asociación Madrileña de ORL, et al. Consenso sobre el diagnóstico y tratamiento de la sordera súbita. Acta Otorrinolaringol Esp. 2011;62:144–57.
3. Herrera M, García Berrocal JR, García Arumí A, et al. Update on consensus on diagnosis and treatment of idiopathic sudden sensorineural hearing loss. Acta Otorrinolaringol Esp (Engl Ed). 2019;70:290–300.
4. Stachler RJ, Chandrasekhar SS, Archer SM, American Academy of Otolaryngology-Head and Neck Surgery, et al. Clinical practice guideline: sudden hearing loss. Otolaryngol Head Neck Surg. 2012;146(3 Suppl):S1–35.

5. Chandrasekhar SS, Tsai Do BS, Schwartz SR, et al. Clinical practice guideline: sudden hearing loss (update). Otolaryngol Head Neck Surg. 2019;161(Suppl. 1):S1–S45.
6. Sauvage JP. Sorderas bruscas y fluctuantes. Enciclopedia Médico-Quirúrgica; 2002. Elsevier, E-20-183-A-10.
7. Narula T, Rennie C. Idiopathic sudden sensorineural hearing loss. In: Watkinson JC, Clarke RW, editors. Scott-Brown's otorhinolaryngology and head and neck surgery. 8th ed. Oxford, UK: CRC Press; 2018. p. 739–51.
8. Chau JK, Lin JR, Atashband S, et al. Systematic review of the evidence for the etiology of adult sudden sensorineural hearing loss. Laryngoscope. 2010;120:1011–21.
9. Herrera Mera M, Santos Duque B, Plaza MG. Etiología de la sordera súbita: no todo es autoinmune. Etiología vascular, infecciosa, por rotura de membranas o de otras causas. In: Plaza G, editor. Sordera súbita: diagnóstico y tratamiento. Madrid: Ergon; 2018. p. 69–92.
10. Gul F, Muderris T, Yalciner G, et al. A comprehensive study of oxidative stress in sudden hearing loss. Eur Arch Otorrinolaringol. 2017;274:1301–8.
11. Hultcrantz E. Sudden deafness—a critical evaluation of pathogenesis and 'cure'. Otorhinolaryngol Nova. 1999;9:178–89.
12. Plontke SK. Diagnostics and therapy of sudden hearing loss. GMS Curr Top Otorhinolaryngol Head Neck Surg. 2017;16:1–21.
13. Yamada S, Kita J, Shinmura D, et al. Update on findings about sudden sensorineural hearing loss and insight into its pathogenesis. J Clin Med. 2022;11:6387.
14. Ballesteros F, Tassies D, Reverter JC, et al. Idiopathic sudden sensorineural hearing loss: classic cardiovascular and new genetic risk factors. Audiol Neurootol. 2012;17:400–8.
15. García-Callejo FJ, Marco-Algarra J, Pla-Gil I, et al. Deformabilidad eritrocitaria patológica en pacientes con sordera súbita. Acta Otorrinolaringol Esp. 2012;63:249–57.
16. García-Callejo FJ, Balaguer-García R, Lis-Sancerni MD, et al. Blood viscosity in COVID-19 patients with sudden deafness. Acta Otorrinolaringol Esp (Engl Ed). 2022;73:104–12.
17. Anderson RG, Meyerhoff WL. Sudden sensorineural hearing loss. Otolaryngol Clin N Am. 1983;16:189–95.
18. Lin RJ, Krall R, Westerberg BD, et al. Systematic review and meta-analysis of the risk factors for sudden sensorineural hearing loss in adults. Laryngoscope. 2012;122:624–35.
19. Kuo CL, Shiao AS, Wang SJ, et al. Risk of sudden sensorineural hearing loss in stroke patients: a 5-year nationwide investigation of 44,460 patients. Medicine (Baltimore). 2016;95:e4841.
20. Kim JY, Hong JY, Kim DK. Association of sudden sensorineural hearing loss with risk of cardiocerebrovascular disease: a study using data from the Korean national health insurance service. JAMA Otolaryngol Head Neck Surg. 2018;144:129–35.
21. Simões JFCPM, Vlaminck S, Seiça RMF, et al. Cardiovascular risk and sudden sensorineural hearing loss: a systematic review and meta-analysis. Laryngoscope. 2023;133:15–24.
22. Saba ES, Swisher AR, Ansari GN, Rivero A. Cardiovascular risk factors in patients with sudden sensorineural hearing loss: a systematic review and meta-analysis. Otolaryngol Head Neck Surg. 2023;168:907–21.
23. Lenkeit CP, Lofgren DH, Zappia J. Cardiovascular risk factors and sudden sensorineural hearing loss: a case-control study. Otol Neurotol. 2023;44:121–5.
24. Mallepally AR, Rustagi T, Chhabra HS, et al. Sensorineural deafness after spine surgery: case series and literature review. World Neurosurg. 2019;131:e482–5.
25. Pau H, Selvadurai D, Murty GE. Reversible sensorineural hearing loss after non-otological surgery under general anaesthetic. Postgrad Med J. 2000;76:304–6.
26. Rhee T, Hwang D, Lee J, et al. Addition of hyperbaric oxygen therapy vs medical therapy alone for idiopathic sudden sensorineural hearing loss: a systematic review and meta-analysis. JAMA Otolaryngol Head Neck Surg. 2018;144:1153–61.
27. Bayoumy AB, Lammet van der Veen E, Alexander de Ru J. Hyperbaric oxygen therapy vs medical therapy for sudden sensorineural hearing loss. JAMA Otolaryngol Head Neck Surg. 2019;145:699–700.
28. Ahn Y, Seo YJ, Lee YS. The effectiveness of hyperbaric oxygen therapy in severe idiopathic sudden sensorineural hearing loss. J Int Adv Otol. 2021;17:215–20.

29. Joshua TG, Ayub A, Wijesinghe P, et al. Hyperbaric oxygen therapy for patients with sudden sensorineural hearing loss: a systematic review and meta-analysis. JAMA Otolaryngol Head Neck Surg. 2022;148:5–11.
30. Mattox DE, Simmons FB. Natural history of sudden sensorineural hearing loss. Ann Otol Rhinol Laryngol. 1977;86:463–80.
31. Wilson WR, Veltri RW, Laird N, et al. Viral and epidemiologic studies of idiopathic sudden hearing loss. Otolaryngol Head Neck Surg. 1983;91:653–8.
32. Gross M, Wolf DG, Elidan J, et al. Enterovirus, cytomegalovirus, and Epstein-Barr virus infection screening in idiopathic sudden sensorineural hearing loss. Audiol Neurootol. 2007;12:179–82.
33. Mishra B, Panda N, Singh MP, et al. Viral infections in sudden hearing loss. Do we have enough evidence? Kathmandu Univ Med J (KUMJ). 2005;3:230–3.
34. Cohen BE, Durstenfeld A, Roehm PC. Viral causes of hearing loss: a review for hearing health professionals. Trends Hear. 2014;18:2331216514541361.
35. Chen X, Fu YY, Zhang TY. Role of viral infection in sudden hearing loss. J Int Med Res. 2019;47:2865–72.
36. López MG, Lanas AV, Albertz NA, et al. Etiología viral de la hipoacusia sensorioneural súbita: ¿Mito o realidad? Rev Otorrinolaringol Cir Cabeza Cuello. 2011;71:215–22.
37. Scalia G, Palermo CI, Maiolino L, et al. Detection of serum IgA to HSV1 and its diagnostic role in sudden hearing loss. New Microbiol. 2013;36:41–7.
38. Park SM, Han C, Lee JW, et al. Does herpes virus reactivation affect prognosis in idiopathic sudden sensorineural hearing loss? Clin Exp Otorhinolaryngol. 2017;10:66–70.
39. Lan WL, Chen CH, Chu YC, et al. Is there an association between concurrent Epstein-Barr virus infection and sudden hearing loss? A case-control study in an East Asian population. J Clin Med. 2023;12:1946.
40. Hughes GB, Freedman MA, Haberkamp TJ, et al. Sudden sensorineural hearing loss. Otolaryngol Clin N Am. 1996;29:393–405.
41. Awad Z, Huins C, Pothier DD. Antivirals for idiopathic sudden sensorineural hearing loss. Cochrane Database Syst Rev. 2012;8:CD006987.
42. García-Berrocal JR, Ramírez-Camacho R, Portero F, et al. Role of viral and Mycoplasma pneumoniae infection in idiopathic sudden sensorineural hearing loss. Acta Otolaryngol. 2000;120:835–59.
43. Espiney Amaro C, Montalvão P, Huins C, et al. Lyme disease: sudden hearing loss as the sole presentation. J Laryngol Otol. 2015;129:183–6.
44. Sowula K, Szaleniec J, Stolcman K, et al. Association between sudden sensorineural hearing loss and lyme disease. J Clin Med. 2021;10(5):1130.
45. Gagnebin J, Maire R. Infection screening in sudden and progressive idiopathic sensorineural hearing loss: a retrospective study of 182 cases. Otol Neurotol. 2002;23:160–2.
46. Cassilde AL, Barnaud G, Baccar S, Mortier E. Sudden-onset bilateral deafness revealing early neurosyphilis. Eur Ann Otorhinolaryngol Head Neck Dis. 2014;131:389–91.
47. McIntyre KM, Favre NM, Kuo CC, Carr MM. Systematic review of sensorineural hearing loss associated with COVID-19 infection. Cureus. 2021;13:e19757.
48. Meng X, Wang J, Sun J, et al. COVID-19 and sudden sensorineural hearing loss: a systematic review. Front Neurol. 2022;13:883749.
49. Pool C, King TS, Pradhan S, et al. Sudden sensorineural hearing loss and coronavirus disease 2019. J Laryngol Otol. 2022;136:823–6.
50. Kaliyappan K, Chen YC, Krishnan Muthaiah VP. Vestibular cochlear manifestations in COVID-19 cases. Front Neurol. 2022;13:850337.
51. Frosolini A, Franz L, Daloiso A, et al. Sudden sensorineural hearing loss in the COVID-19 pandemic: a systematic review and meta-analysis. Diagnostics (Basel). 2022;12:3139.
52. Fancello V, Fancello G, Hatzopoulos S, et al. Sensorineural hearing loss post-COVID-19 infection: an update. Audiol Res. 2022;12:307–15.
53. Chari DA, Parikh A, Kozin ED, et al. Impact of COVID-19 on presentation of sudden sensorineural hearing loss at a single institution. Otolaryngol Head Neck Surg. 2021;165:163–5.

54. van Rijssen LB, Derks W, Hoffmans R, et al. No COVID-19 in patients with sudden sensori-neural hearing loss (SSNHL). Otol Neurotol. 2022;43:170–3.
55. Doweck I, Yanir Y, Najjar-Debbiny R, et al. Sudden sensorineural hearing loss during the COVID-19 pandemic. JAMA Otolaryngol Head Neck Surg. 2022;148:373–5.
56. Hafrén L, Saarinen R, Lundberg M. Effects of social distancing on the incidence of Bell's palsy and sudden sensorineural hearing loss. Acta Otolaryngol. 2022;142:220–3.
57. Yanir Y, Doweck I, Shibli R, et al. Association between the BNT162b2 messenger RNA COVID-19 vaccine and the risk of sudden sensorineural hearing loss. JAMA Otolaryngol Head Neck Surg. 2022;148:299–306.
58. Formeister EJ, Wu MJ, Chari DA, et al. Assessment of sudden sensorineural hearing loss after COVID-19 vaccination. JAMA Otolaryngol Head Neck Surg. 2022;148:307–15.
59. Ulrich AK, Sundaram ME, Osterholm MT. Rare sudden sensorineural hearing loss potentially associated with COVID-19 vaccination does not outweigh the benefit of COVID-19 vaccines. JAMA Otolaryngol Head Neck Surg. 2022;148:315–6.
60. Pisani D, Gioacchini FM, Viola P, et al. Audiovestibular disorders after COVID-19 vaccine: is there an association? Audiol Res. 2022;12:212–23.
61. Nieminen TA, Kivekäs I, Artama M, et al. Sudden hearing loss following vaccination against COVID-19. JAMA Otolaryngol Head Neck Surg. 2023;149:133–40.
62. Fisher R, Tarnovsky Y, Hirshoren N, et al. The association between COVID-19 vaccination and idiopathic sudden sensorineural hearing loss, clinical manifestation and outcomes. Eur Arch Otorrinolaringol. 2023;280(8):3609–13. https://doi.org/10.1007/s00405-023-07869-2.
63. Cohen Michael O, Tamir SO, O'Rourke N, Marom T. Audiometry-confirmed sudden sensori-neural hearing loss incidence among COVID-19 patients and BNT162b2 vaccine recipients. Otol Neurotol. 2023;44:e68–72.
64. Damkier P, Cleary B, Hallas J, et al. Sudden sensorineural hearing loss following immuniza-tion with BNT162b2 or mRNA-1273: a Danish population-based cohort study. Otolaryngol Head Neck Surg. 2023;169(6):1472–80. https://doi.org/10.1002/ohn.394.
65. Albakri K, Abdelwahab OA, Gabra MD, et al. Characteristics of sudden hearing loss after different COVID-19 vaccinations: a systematic review and meta-analysis. Eur Arch Otorrinolaringol. 2023;280(12):5167–76.
66. Goodhill V. Labyrinthine membrane ruptures in sudden sensorineural hearing loss. Proc R Soc Med. 1976;69:565–72.
67. Nagai T, Nagai M. Labyrinthine window rupture as a cause of acute sensorineural hearing loss. Eur Arch Otorrinolaringol. 2012;269:67–71.
68. Kampfner D, Anagiotos A, Luers JC, et al. Analysis of 101 patients with severe to profound sudden unilateral hearing loss treated with explorative tympanotomy and sealing of the round window membrane. Eur Arch Otorrinolaringol. 2014;271:2145–52.
69. Loader B, Seemann R, Atteneder C, et al. Sealing of the round and oval window niches with triamcinolone-soaked fascia as salvage surgical therapy in sudden sensorineural hearing loss. Acta Otolaryngol. 2017;137:923–7.
70. Lou Z, Lou Z. Surgical indications or inclusion/exclusion criteria of explorative tympanotomy on sudden sensorineural hearing. Am J Otolaryngol. 2018;39(3):365–6.
71. Prenzler NK, Schwab B, Kaplan DM, et al. The role of explorative tympanotomy in patients with sudden sensorineural hearing loss with and without perilymphatic fistula. Am J Otolaryngol. 2018;39:46–9.
72. Thomas JP, Drewermann S, Voelter C, et al. Prognostic factors regarding the hearing outcome in severe to profound sudden sensorineural hearing loss treated by tympanotomy and seal-ing of labyrinthine windows after ineffective systemic corticosteroid application. Eur Arch Otorrinolaringol. 2018;275:1749–58.
73. Heilen S, Lang CP, Warnecke A, et al. Exploratory tympanotomy in sudden sensorineural hear-ing loss for the identification of a perilymphatic fistula-retrospective analysis and review of the literature. J Laryngol Otol. 2020;134:501–8.

74. Chen N, Karpeta N, Ma X, et al. Diagnosis, differential diagnosis, and treatment for sudden sensorineural hearing loss: current otolaryngology practices in China. Front Neurol. 2023;14:1121324.
75. Thielker J, Heuschkel A, Boeger D, et al. Patients with non-idiopathic sudden sensorineural hearing loss show hearing improvement more often than patients with idiopathic sensorineural hearing loss. Eur Arch Otorrinolaringol. 2022;279:663–75.
76. Tsuzuki N, Wasano K. Idiopathic sudden sensorineural hearing loss: A review focused on the contribution of vascular pathologies. Auris Nasus Larynx. 2024;51(4):747–54.

Diagnostic Assessment and Complementary Tests in Sudden Sensorineural Hearing Loss

Concepción Rodríguez Izquierdo,
Mar Martínez Ruiz-Coello, and Guillermo Plaza

Concept

Sudden hearing loss (SHL) is the rapid onset of the sensation of hearing loss in one or both ears [1–3]; sudden sensorineural hearing loss is a subtype of sensorineural hearing loss that occurs in less than 72 h and requires the fulfilment of certain audiometric criteria defined in the published consensus [2–5] and idiopathic sudden sensorineural hearing loss (ISSNHL) is when the cause is not identified [3–5].

The diagnosis of SSNHL is by definition a diagnosis of exclusion, and the initial examination of the patient should rule out other causes of sensorineural hearing loss. Once SSNHL has been confirmed, approximately 90% of cases are idiopathic. The remaining 10% are usually related to retrocochlear pathology (neurinoma, multiple sclerosis, etc.) [6–10].

SSNHL is a true neuro-otological urgency as the possibility of hearing recovery decreases with the delay in starting treatment as most case series have shown [11–13]. Since this is an urgent situation of a not very well-known nature, uncertain clinical course and prognosis, it is necessary to establish three fundamental lines of action for its correct management:

1. Information and education on ISSNHL for patients, giving increasing importance to telemedicine and computer applications.

C. Rodríguez Izquierdo (✉)
Ear, Nose and Throat Department, Hospital Universitario de Fuenlabrada, Madrid, Spain

M. Martínez Ruiz-Coello
Ear, Nose and Throat Department, Hospital Clínico San Carlos, Madrid, Spain

G. Plaza
Ear, Nose and Throat Department, Hospital Universitario de Fuenlabrada, Madrid, Spain

Ear, Nose and Throat Department, Hospital Universitario Sanitas La Zarzuela, Madrid, Spain

Universidad Rey Juan Carlos, Madrid, Spain

G. Plaza, J. R. García Berrocal (eds.), *Sudden Sensorineural Hearing Loss*,
https://doi.org/10.1007/978-3-031-61385-2_4

2. ISSNHL training for GPs and A&E doctors, with the aim of reducing diagnostic delay.
3. Establishment of an evidence-based diagnostic-therapeutic protocol for ISSNHL in ENT services.

It is important to remember that, in most cases, the patient is not always seen in the first instance by the ENT doctor, but instead goes to the A&E or to their GP [11]. Therefore, it is necessary to include these general health points of care in the diagnostic protocol [14, 15]. Avoiding the implication of GPs and A&E will result in failure to approach SSNHL.

Role of the Patient and Telemedicine in the Diagnosis of SSNHL

As emphasised in the North American consensus, patients need to be aware of the importance of SSNHL [5]. When they notice a significant difference in hearing in both ears, they should try to get an appointment with a doctor as soon as possible. Unfortunately, many times this is not the case, and they go to their doctor days later, or even weeks later than the onset of symptoms. Only by making this condition known will we get them to visit their doctor as soon as possible.

American literature places a lot of screening-related value on the so-called *hum test*, in which the patient is asked to hum to see whether they hear the hum differently in the deaf ear and in the healthy ear [1, 16]. Patients should be informed of this tool.

Computer science and its application to telecommunications are playing an ever-growing role in medical care and contribute to the development of new branches of medicine such as telemedicine and teleassistance, which were fundamental during the COVID-19 pandemic. For example, the Massachusetts General Hospital website devotes space to information and education on SSNHL for patients, even giving telephone numbers for assistance by nurses (http://www.masseyeandear.org/for-patients/patient-guide/patienteducation/diseases-and-conditions/sudden-deafness).

In the near future, the development of this type of care may acquire more prominence in the management of certain processes and perhaps also ISSNHL [17–19]. Thus, the use by patients themselves of audiometric tests with validated smartphone apps could help with an earlier diagnosis through telemedicine (Fig. 1).

For instance, during the COVID-19 pandemic, Shilo et al. [20] developed an SSNHL diagnostic programme with the support of telemedicine. The patients, trained in the above-mentioned *hum test* and using a *smartphone* audiometry exam, achieved an SSNHL self-diagnostic reliability of 84%.

Undoubtedly, outreach campaigns in the general population are crucial. For example, the Spanish Society of Otorhinolaryngology and Head & Neck Surgery (SEORL-CCC) has published press releases and videos to provide information on ISSNHL to the general public. It would be interesting to design strategies of scientific dissemination about this condition in primary care through professional scientific societies.

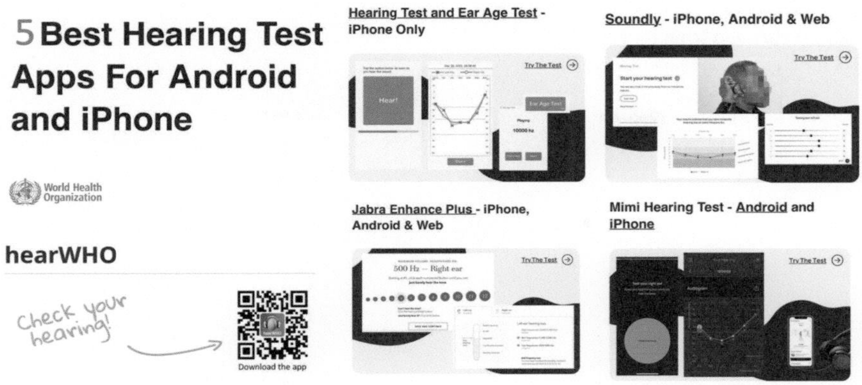

5 Best Hearing Test Apps For Android and iPhone

World Health Organization

hearWHO

Check your hearing!

Download the app

Hearing Test and Ear Age Test - iPhone Only

Soundly - iPhone, Android & Web

Jabra Enhance Plus - iPhone, Android & Web

Mimi Hearing Test - Android and iPhone

Fig. 1 Best audiometric app for smartphones. Four of them are recommended at https://www. soundly.com/blog/hearing-test-apps. WHO recommends its own: https://www.who.int/teams/ noncommunicable-diseases/sensory-functions-disability-and-rehabilitation/hearwho

Role of GPS and A&E Doctors in the Diagnosis of SSNHL

Once the patient suspects that they have SSNHL, it is most common for them to go to A&E or their GP. At this level, the non-specialist doctor has the fundamental mission of establishing the diagnosis by ruling out SSNHL with the means at their disposal [14, 15, 21]:

- Anamnesis: Aimed at confirming the suspicion of hearing loss, ruling out the existence of associated symptoms such as tinnitus or vertigo and asking about previous trauma, pain in the ear canal, discharge, fever and other associated symptoms that justify hearing loss.
- Otoscopy: Aimed at viewing the tympanic membrane to rule out pathology of the external and middle ear. If cerumen is present, it should be removed and the examination completed.
- Acoumetry (tuning forks): The Weber test is the screening test par excellence [22]. It is conducted by placing the 256 or 512 Hz tuning fork on the vertex or on the incisors of the patient's upper jaw (Fig. 2). The patient is then asked where they can hear the sound; it is normal to obtain an indifferent result, while suspected SSNHL always lateralises towards the healthy ear, becoming a very reliable predictor [1, 3, 7, 23].

With these three tools, the GP or A&E doctor should be able to confirm the suspicion of SSNHL. The truth is that the availability and knowledge of the use of tuning forks in primary care is an issue to be improved as observed in two recent Canadian and British surveys [24, 25], where more than 40% of GPs do not have access to tuning forks.

Fig. 2 Acoumetry (tuning forks): Weber and Rinne tests

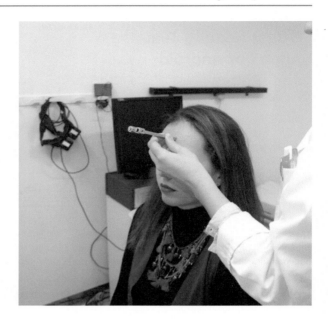

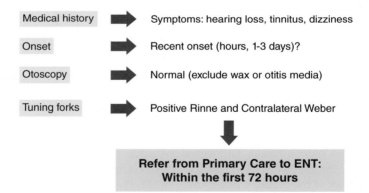

Fig. 3 Diagnostic algorithm for primary care for SSNHL to refer the patient urgently to the ENT specialist. (Modified from Muñoz-Proto et al. [13])

Therefore, in order to reduce the delay until the start of treatment, it is essential to involve GPs, raising their awareness to determine whether the case in question is SSNHL or not, as evidenced in the protocol defended by Muñoz-Proto et al. for primary care [15] (Fig. 3).

Role of Specialised Care in the Diagnosis of SSNHL

Once the patient suspected of having SSNHL is referred to an ENT specialist, the ENT specialist must confirm the SSNHL symptoms and rule out any underlying causes before diagnosing SSNHL or not, and this must be done as soon as possible [3, 5].

To confirm the SSNHL diagnosis, it is necessary to carry out a thorough anamnesis and perform audiological tests following the *American National Standards* or those recognised by the Spanish Association of Audiology (2002) [26, 27].

In all cases, to confirm the SSNHL diagnosis and determine its prognosis, audiological tests should include

- Pure tone audiometry (PTA): Diagnosis is established with a loss of >30 dB in three consecutive frequencies. Audiograms can have prognostic implications; when low frequencies are affected, they respond better to treatment (Fig. 4.4a), whereas if high and especially pantonal frequencies are affected (Fig. 4.4b, c), they evolve worse.
- Speech audiometry: The speech recognition threshold (SRT) is detected and the maximum discrimination test (MaxDT) is performed with masking on the healthy ear. SRT and MaxDT let the specialist check the results of the PTA, assess whether the process is cochlear or retrocochlear and report on the degree of hearing impairment.
- Impedance audiometry:
  - Tympanometry, to determine the normality of the middle ear, excluding frequent pathologies such as otitis media with effusion or Eustachian tube dysfunction.
  - Detection of contralateral and ipsilateral stapedial reflex (SR) thresholds, from 500 to 4000 Hz, including the Metz test, to rule out the presence of cochlear recruitment. Gerwin and LaCosta [28] described that the existence of stapedial reflex is a factor of good prognosis of SSNHL.

However, with the diagnostic confirmation of SSNHL by PTA, quantification of damage by speech audiometry and topographic guidance by impedance measurement, the diagnosis that the ENT specialist must make does not end there, as it is still possible to further explore aetiological background through a complete clinical history.

In a full anamnesis carried out by the ENT specialist, it is essential to rule out family history of genetic diseases; personal history of otitis; trauma; rheumatological, neurological, cardiovascular, oncological and endocrinological (diabetes) processes; pregnancies; surgeries and even exposure to ototoxic drugs.

Regarding symptoms, the sensation of ear fullness, which precedes hearing loss, is typical, as is the coexistence of tinnitus in 70% of cases and vertigo in up to 50% of cases.

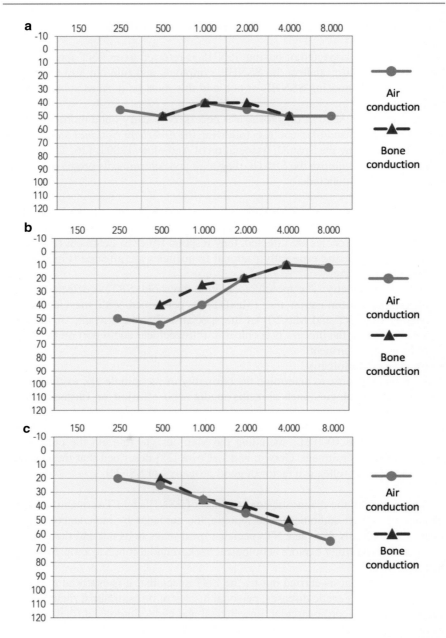

Fig. 4.4 (**a**) Audiogram. SSNHL with hearing loss in all frequencies (pantonal). (**b**) Audiogram. SSNHL with hearing loss only in low frequencies. (**c**) Audiogram. SSNHL with hearing loss only in high frequencies (acute SSNHL)

In patients with recurrent or fluctuating episodes of SSNHL, causes such as Ménière's disease, autoimmune diseases of the inner ear, Cogan's syndrome and hyperviscosity syndromes should be suspected.

When SSNHL is accompanied by neurological focality, the specialist should rule out central nervous system-related pathology, such as cerebrovascular accidents (CVAs), due to the involvement of the anterior inferior cerebellar artery (AICA), multiple sclerosis or neoplastic meningitis.

Within bilateral SSNHL, the groups of simultaneous SSNHL (the second ear is affected in a space of time <72 h) and sequential SSNHL (the second ear is affected in a space of time >72 h) can be included as they correspond to variants of the same syndromes with a poor auditory prognosis [29–31].

Complementary Tests in the Diagnosis of SSNHL

Laboratory Tests

There is little evidence that a routine series of analytical tests influences the management of SSNHL. In fact, the North American consensus on SSNHL indicates that it should not be requested [4, 5].

However, the alteration of certain analytical parameters (ESR, PCR, antinuclear antibodies, serology of syphilis, etc.) could point to an underlying cause, while certain tests such as the request for *B. burgdorferi* titres in endemic regions may be effective.

Numerous biomarkers have been associated with ISSNHL [32–37]. Of particular note are fibrinogen (the higher the level, the worse the prognosis) and whose increase points to a vascular aetiology due to an increase in blood viscosity [38–40]; neutrophil–lymphocyte ratio (the higher the level, the worse the prognosis) and whose increase is associated with an inflammatory aetiology [41, 42]; the concentration of C-reactive protein and cytokines such as TNF alpha, IL-1 and others, whose increase is related to inflammatory aetiology [34, 35]; and, finally, prestin (a cochlear protein), whose presence in the blood denotes early cochlear damage [43, 44]. The study of these factors is of prognostic interest and currently the subject of various research papers.

In the current Spanish consensus on SSNHL, it is recommended to request a basic analysis with blood count, biochemistry and ANA in all cases [2, 3].

Diagnostic Radiology

In all patients with SSNHL, it is essential to rule out the presence of retrocochlear pathology. The gold standard technique is magnetic resonance imaging (MRI) with high-resolution *fast spin echo* sequences of the internal auditory canal (IAC), which offers better results and lower costs than gadolinium MRI [11].

The biggest drawback is that this technique is not available in all care settings. In cases where it is contraindicated or when it is not readily available, brainstem auditory-evoked potentials (BAEPs) or serial PTA can be performed [3, 11].

In addition, MRI has the added advantage of being able to identify other causes of SSNHL (cochlear inflammation or MS) or findings that involve some underlying aetiology (cerebral small vessel disease) [45] (see chapter "MRI in Sudden Sensorineural Hearing").

Therefore, in the current Spanish consensus on SSNHL, it is recommended to request an MRI in all cases of SSNHL, with it ideally being performed in the first 2 weeks after diagnosis (Fig. 4.5) [2, 3, 11].

Other Audiological Tests

The ENT specialist has access to a series of audio-vestibular tests that can complete the diagnosis of SSNHL and guide the prognosis individually.

Otoacoustic emissions (OAEs) are based on sounds emitted by the cochlea as a result of the activity of the external hair cells of the organ of Corti, which protrude outwards and can be detected in the external auditory canal. There are different types of OAE:

- Spontaneous otoacoustic emissions (SOAEs): These are OAEs that occur in the absence of stimulus. They are only recorded in 50% of ears with normal hearing and in few frequencies, so their clinical usefulness is limited.
- Transient-evoked OAEs (TEOAEs): Produced by a brief stimulus (click, tone burst, etc.). Indicated for the detection of cochlear lesions and especially in the early diagnosis of hearing loss.
- Evoked otoacoustic emissions (EOAEs): These are OAEs that are generated in response to a sound stimulus. They are recorded in most normal ears.

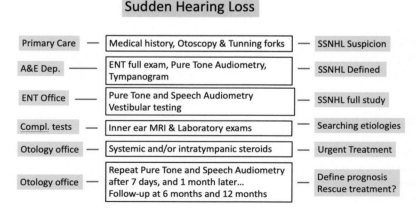

Fig. 4.5 Diagnostic/therapeutic algorithm for ISSNHL [11]

- Distortion products (DP): Produced by stimulation with two simulated pure tones, which results in the emission of a third tone with a different frequency from the frequencies of the tones used as a stimulus. They are clinically useful as they allow the frequent study and early detection of mild cochlear damage not observable with conventional audiometry.

The study of OAEs may have a prognostic interest for ISSNHL [40–44]. Nakamura et al. [46] performed OAEs, TEOAEs and DP in 15 patients with ISSNHL, observing that the amplitude of the three forms of OAE increased as there was a hearing improvement, and that the OAEs recovered when said improvement occurred, demonstrating a functional recovery of the external hair cells. Chao and Chen [47], Liu et al. [48], El-Sayed et al. [49] and Subirana et al. [50] studied DP as a prognostic factor of ISSNHL, observing that, if they have greater amplitude, ISSNHL improves.

In addition to their diagnostic role to rule out retrocochlear pathology, **auditory-evoked potentials (AEPs)** have prognostic interest. Wang et al. [51] found a correlation between the presence of AEP registration and hearing improvement, with the presence of a wave in the AEP being the most relevant prognostic factor for these authors.

Electrocochleography (ECoG) is a recording of an electrophysiological event that takes place in the cochlea after an acoustic stimulus. The EcoG recording consists mainly of two pre-synthetic components, the cochlear microphysical potential and the summation potential (SP), and a post-synthetic component, which is the compound action potential (CAP). Since the SP wave is generated by the hair cells, its amplitude is considerably decreased in sensorineural hearing loss. In contrast, the CAP represents the sum of the responses of thousands of fibres of the auditory nerve that are discharged simultaneously. A widely used clinical ratio is the SP/CAP ratio.

Junicho et al. [52] presented a case series of 184 patients with low-frequency ISSNHL that were compared with patients with high-frequency ISSNHL and patients diagnosed with Ménière's disease. EcoG was performed on all of them, observing how the presence of vertigo at the diagnosis of ISSNHL and an altered EcoG recording in ISSNHL correlate with a higher recurrence rate of deafness and with a progression to Ménière's disease. In fact, the mean values of the SP/CAP ratio were similar between cases of recurrent ISSNHL and cases of Ménière's disease.

Fushiki et al. [53] published a paper on ISSNHL, differentiating cases with high- or low-frequency involvement and observing their evolution at 4 years. In a sample of 61 patients, they observed that the recurrence rate of ISSNHL was 20% after 1 year and 43% after 5 years in low-frequency ISSNHL, compared to 12% and 31%, respectively, in high-frequency ISSNHL.

Recently, the interest of EcoG has led to the prediction and confirmation of the diagnosis of Ménière's disease. Hornibrook et al. [54] published a paper in which the findings in MRI and EcoG provided the diagnosis of this disease with considerable certainty.

Other Vestibular Tests

The main interest here lies in ruling out the diagnosis of vestibular neuritis, making a differential diagnosis with Ménière's disease and serving as tools with prognostic value of ISSNHL itself.

With regard to **electronystagmography (ENG)**, Junicho et al. [55] studied patients with ISSNHL who underwent ENG and glycerol tests, observing how many patients evolved to Ménière's disease. In those in which upward-sloping hearing loss predominated, the presence of spontaneous nystagmus in the ENG recording appeared in half of the cases, although they did not suffer from vertigo, and it was associated with progression to Ménière's disease in 15% of cases. Cho et al. [56] studied calorie tests and MRI images in a case series of 200 patients with SSNHL. In the 25 patients in whom MRI showed specific causes of SSNHL (schwannomas or intralabyrinthine haemorrhages), canal paresis was more frequent.

Vestibular myogenic-evoked potentials (VEMPs) are based on the study of the vestibular-cervical or vestibular-ocular reflex that is triggered by static stimulation. The response to the stimulus is a potential for inhibitory action in the sternocleido-mastoid muscle on the same side of the stimulated ear (cVEMPs) or excitatory in the lower oblique muscle (III pair) on the opposite side of the stimulated ear (oVEMPs). The said response is collected, analysed electronically and automatically portrayed in a graph. For its valuation, it is useful to compare the two ears, with an asymmetry greater than 30% being considered abnormal. CVEMPs, which measure the activity of the saccule-spinal pathway (inferior vestibular nerve), or oVEMPs, which collect the activation of the utricle-ocular pathway (superior vestibular nerve), can be performed.

The value of VEMPs in ISSNHL has been studied by several authors [11, 57–60]. Hong et al. [57] described that the absence of VEMPs is associated with more profound and worse prognostic ISSNHL. In her doctoral thesis, Dra. Genestar Bosch defined, in a sample of 73 patients with ISSNHL, that the presence of normal VEMPs is associated with a higher probability of hearing recovery [58]. Niu et al. [59] observed that the absence of normal recVEMPs and oVEMPs and altered caloric tests result in a lower probability of hearing improvement.

Belonging to the Halmagyi group, Pogson et al. [61] used the **video head impulse test (vHIT)** and VEMPS to study 37 patients with ISSNHL. They found that 74% of the patients had an altered posterior semicircular canal, differentiating these cases from vestibular neuritis in which the involvement of the horizontal and upper channels is more frequent. Battat et al. [62] also studied vHIT in ISSNHL, showing that the site of insult in patients with ISSNHL without true vertigo is usually limited to the cochlea or the cochlear nerve.

Fujimoto et al. [63] published a similar paper on 25 patients, once again verifying that the alteration in cVEMPs, oVEMPSs and caloric tests has a prognostic meaning, but adding that it also has a localising capacity of the origin of the lesion, with a worse prognosis when there is involvement of the utricle.

In the same sense, Oiticica et al. [64] studied the usefulness of OAEs by means of DP, VEMPs, caloric tests and MRI. The authors insist that this series of tests makes it possible to reach a functional diagnosis of each case of ISSNHL.

Similarly, Lee et al. [65] observed that the greater the audiovestibular involvement, the worse the prognosis will be, especially when it affects the superior vestibular nerve, and established four types of ISSNHL:

- ISSNHL with cVEMPS and normal caloric tests: pure cochlear damage (C).
- ISSNHL with normal cVEMPS, but altered caloric tests: cochlear and superior vestibular damage (C + S).
- ISSNHL with altered cVEMPS and normal caloric tests: cochlear and inferior vestibular damage (C + I).
- ISSNHL with cVEMPS and altered caloric tests: cochlear, superior vestibular and inferior vestibular damage (C + S + I).

Finally, in the recent meta-analysis by Yu et al. [66], the 18 most relevant papers on vestibular testing in ISSNHL were reviewed (Fig. 4.6). According to this paper, the most frequently damaged vestibular organ in ISSNHL is the utricle and upper semicircular canal (U + S). If the patient suffers from vertigo in the course of ISSNHL, they have an OR of 4.89 (95% CI: 1.2–19.9) for vestibular involvement, and in this case, their probability of hearing recovery is lower, with an OR of 0.24 (95% CI: 0.11–0.5).

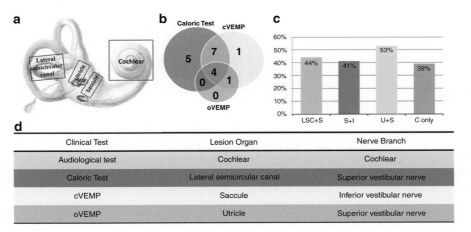

Fig. 4.6 Topographic diagnosis in ISSNHL by means of audiovestibular tests. (**a**) Schematic diagram of the vestibulocochlear lesion patterns, including the cochlea, saccule, utricle and lateral semicircular canal. (**b**) Distributions of vestibular test abnormalities of all 18 studies, including 16 by caloric test, 13 by cervical vestibular-evoked myogenic potential test (cVEMP) and 5 by ocular vestibular-evoked myogenic potential test (oVEMP). (**c**) Percentage of inner ear lesion locations in the included studies—LSC + S, abnormal caloric test; S + I, abnormal cVEMP test; U + S, abnormal oVEMP test; and C only, cochlear impairment only. (**d**) Table of clinical tests performed, organs involved, and their corresponding innervation. (From Yu et al. [66])

Similarly, Kizkapan et al. [67], Castellucci et al. [68], Hong et al. [69] and Shen et al. [70] have also shown that studying the vestibular profile has prognostic value in ISSNHL, also helping to differentiate between ischemia and viral cochleitis. Therefore, the ENT specialist should be encouraged to use complementary audio-vestibular testing to help determine the prognosis of each patient with ISSNHL [65–72].

Conclusions

SSNHL is a neuro-otological emergency with uncertain prognosis and irreversible consequences in many cases. Most cases are treated by A&E doctors in the first instance. As has been seen in the pandemic, telemedicine will facilitate the participation of patients themselves in the diagnosis of SSNHL. With a suspected diagnosis, patients are referred to the ENT specialist for audiological evaluation with pure tone audiometry, speech audiometry and tympanometry, which end up confirming it. The presence of retrocochlear pathology should be ruled out with MRI. Other audiovestibular tests are helpful in completing the diagnosis of ISSNHL and establishing prognosis. It is important to assess the balance of each patient, rule out vestibular neuritis and make a differential diagnosis with Ménière's disease to offer more information on the prognosis.

References

1. Rauch SD. Clinical practice. Idiopathic sudden sensorineural hearing loss. N Engl J Med. 2008;359:833–40.
2. Plaza G, Durio E, Herráiz C, Asociación Madrileña de ORL, et al. Consenso sobre el diagnóstico y tratamiento de la sordera súbita. Acta Otorrinolaringol Esp. 2011;62:144–57.
3. Herrera M, García Berrocal JR, García Arumí A, et al. Update on consensus on diagnosis and treatment of idiopathic sudden sensorineural hearing loss. Acta Otorrinolaringol Esp (Engl Ed). 2019;70:290–300.
4. Stachler RJ, Chandrasekhar SS, Archer SM, American Academy of Otolaryngology-Head and Neck Surgery, et al. Clinical practice guideline: sudden hearing loss. Otolaryngol Head Neck Surg. 2012;146(Suppl. 3):S1–35.
5. Chandrasekhar SS, Tsai Do BS, Schwartz SR, et al. Clinical practice guideline: sudden hearing loss (update). Otolaryngol Head Neck Surg. 2019;161(Suppl. 1):S1–S45.
6. Narula T, Rennie C. Idiopathic sudden sensorineural hearing loss. In: Watkinson JC, Clarke RW, editors. Scott-Brown's otorhinolaryngology and head and neck surgery. 8th ed. Oxford, UK: CRC Press; 2018. p. 739–51.
7. Plontke SK. Diagnostics and therapy of sudden hearing loss. GMS Curr Top Otorhinolaryngol Head Neck Surg. 2017;16:1–21.
8. Chau JK, Lin JR, Atashband S, et al. Systematic review of the evidence for the etiology of adult sudden sensorineural hearing loss. Laryngoscope. 2010;120(5):1011–21.
9. Herrera Mera M, Santos Duque B, Plaza MG. Etiología de la sordera súbita: no todo es autoinmune. Etiología vascular, infecciosa, por rotura de membranas o de otras causas. In: Plaza G, editor. Sordera súbita: diagnóstico y tratamiento. Madrid: Ergon; 2018. p. 69–92.

10. Thielker J, Heuschkel A, Boeger D, et al. Patients with non-idiopathic sudden sensorineural hearing loss show hearing improvement more often than patients with idiopathic sudden sensorineural hearing loss. Eur Arch Otorrinolaringol. 2022;279(2):663–75.

11. Plaza G. Sordera súbita: diagnóstico y tratamiento. Madrid: Ergon; 2018.

12. Jung WW, Hoegerl C. Sudden sensorineural hearing loss and why it's an emergency. Cureus. 2022;14(1):e21418.

13. Klein L, Handzel O, Shilo S, et al. Is sudden sensorineural hearing loss an otologic emergency? evidence-based cutoff for optimal treatment initiation for sudden unilateral sensorineural hearing loss: a case series and meta-analyses. Otol Neurotol. 2023;44:216–22.

14. Morales Salas M, Ventura DJ. Hipoacusia brusca: aproximación diagnóstica y terapéutica. SEMERGEN. 2000;26:458–62.

15. Muñoz-Proto F, Carnevale C, Bejarano-Panadés N. Manejo de hipoacusia neurosensorial súbita en atención primaria. SEMERGEN. 2014;40:149–54.

16. Ahmed OH, Gallant SC, Ruiz R, et al. Validity of the hum test, a simple and reliable alternative to the Weber test. Ann Otol Rhinol Laryngol. 2018;127:402–5.

17. Lin HH, Chu YC, Lai YH, et al. A smartphone-based approach to screening for sudden sensorineural hearing loss: cross-sectional validity study. JMIR Mhealth Uhealth. 2020;8(11):e23047.

18. Hazan A, Luberadzka J, Rivilla J, et al. Home-based audiometry with a smartphone app: reliable results? Am J Audiol. 2022;31:914–22.

19. Chen CH, Lin HH, Wang MC, et al. Diagnostic accuracy of smartphone-based audiometry for hearing loss detection: meta-analysis. JMIR Mhealth Uhealth. 2021;9:e28378.

20. Shilo S, Ungar OJ, Handzel O, et al. Telemedicine for patients with unilateral sudden hearing loss in the COVID-19 era. JAMA Otolaryngol Head Neck Surg. 2022;148:166–72.

21. Ojha S, Henderson A, Bennett W, Clark M. Sudden sensorineural hearing loss and bedside phone testing: a guide for primary care. Br J Gen Pract. 2020;70:144–5.

22. Shuman AG, Li X, Halpin CF, et al. Tuning fork testing in sudden sensorineural hearing loss. JAMA Intern Med. 2013;173:706–7.

23. Kelly EA, Li B, Adams ME. Diagnostic accuracy of tuning fork tests for hearing loss: a systematic review. Otolaryngol Head Neck Surg. 2018;159:220–30.

24. Ng B, Crowson MG, Lin V. Management of sudden sensorineural hearing loss among primary care physicians in Canada: a survey study. J Otolaryngol Head Neck Surg. 2021;50:22.

25. Embury-Young Y, Shelton F, Clamp P. Assessing sudden onset hearing loss in general practice: where are the tuning forks? Clin Otolaryngol. 2023;48(6):925–8.

26. AEDA. Normalización de las pruebas Audiológicas (I): la audiometría tonal liminar [en línea]. Auditio: Rev Electrón Audiol. 2002;1:16–9.

27. AEDA. Normalización de las pruebas audiológicas (II): La audiometría verbal o logoaudiometría [en linea]. Auditio: Rev Electrón Audiol. 2002;1:34–6.

28. Gerwin JM, LaCoste P. The acoustic stapedial reflex as a prognostic indicator in sudden onset sensorineural hearing loss. Otolaryngol Head Neck Surg. 1982;90:857–61.

29. Sara SA, Teh BM, Friedland P. Bilateral sudden sensorineural hearing loss: review. J Laryngol Otol. 2014;128(Suppl. 1):S8–15.

30. Elias TGA, Monsanto RDC, Jean LS, et al. Bilateral sudden sensorineural hearing loss: a distinct phenotype entity. Otol Neurotol. 2022;43:437–42.

31. Wang Y, Xiong W, Sun X, et al. Characteristics and prognosis analysis of bilateral sudden sensorineural hearing loss: a retrospective case-control study. Clin Otolaryngol. 2022;47:732–40.

32. Doo JG, Kim D, Kim Y, et al. Biomarkers suggesting favorable prognostic outcomes in sudden sensorineural hearing loss. Int J Mol Sci. 2020;21:7248.

33. Frosolini A, Franz L, Daloiso A, et al. Digging into the role of inflammatory biomarkers in sudden sensorineural hearing loss diagnosis and prognosis: a systematic review and meta-analysis. Medicina (Kaunas). 2022;58:963.

34. Diao T, Ke Y, Zhang J, et al. Correlation between the prognosis of sudden total deafness and the peripheral blood inflammation markers. Front Neurol. 2022;13:927235.

35. Chen L, Wang M, Zhang W, et al. The value of inflammatory biomarkers in the occurrence and prognosis of sudden sensorineural hearing loss: a meta-analysis. Eur Arch Otorrinolaringol. 2023;280:3119–29.
36. Al-Azzawi A, Stapleton E. Blood tests as biomarkers for the diagnosis and prognosis of sudden sensorineural hearing loss in adults: a systematic review. J Laryngol Otol. 2023;137:977–84.
37. Niknazar S, Bazgir N, Shafaei V, et al. Assessment of prognostic biomarkers in sudden sensorineural hearing loss: a systematic review and meta-analysis. Clin Biochem. 2023;121–122:110684.
38. Oya R, Takenaka Y, Imai T, et al. Serum fibrinogen as a prognostic factor in sudden sensorineural hearing loss: a meta-analysis. Otol Neurotol. 2018;39:e929–5.
39. Okuda H, Aoki M, Ohashi T, et al. Serum fibrinogen level and cytokine production as prognostic biomarkers for idiopathic sudden sensorineural hearing loss. Otol Neurotol. 2022;43:e712–9.
40. Weiss BG, Spiegel JL, Becker S, et al. Randomized, placebo-controlled study on efficacy, safety and tolerability of drug-induced defibrinogenation for sudden sensorineural hearing loss: the lessons learned. Eur Arch Otorrinolaringol. 2023;280:4009–18.
41. Kang JW, Kim MG, Kim SS, et al. Neutrophil-lymphocyte ratio as a valuable prognostic marker in idiopathic sudden sensorineural hearing loss. Acta Otolaryngol. 2020;140:307–13.
42. Ni W, Song SP, Jiang YD. Association between routine hematological parameters and sudden sensorineural hearing loss: a meta-analysis. J Otol. 2021;16:47–54.
43. Iliadou E, Kikidis D, Pastiadis K, et al. Blood prestin levels in normal hearing and in sensorineural hearing loss: a scoping review. Ear Hear. 2021;42:1127–36.
44. Saadat F, Jalali MM, Akbari M. Assessment of prestin level changes as an inner-ear biomarker in patients with idiopathic sudden sensorineural hearing loss. J Laryngol Otol. 2022;136:1039–43.
45. Covelli E, Filippi C, Elfarargy HH, et al. The impact of labyrinthine magnetic resonance signal alterations on the treatment of sudden sensory-neural hearing loss. Acta Otolaryngol. 2023;143:459–65.
46. Nakamura M, Yamasoba T, Kaga K. Changes in otoacoustic emissions in patients with idiopathic sudden deafness. Audiology. 1997;36:121–35.
47. Chao TK, Chen TH. Distortion product otoacoustic emissions as a prognostic factor for idiopathic sudden sensorineural hearing loss. Audiol Neurootol. 2006;11:331–8.
48. Liu SY, Shi WY, Zheng HY, et al. The correlation between detection value of distortion-product otoacoustic emissions and the early prognosis of sudden sensorineural hearing Loss. J Int Adv Otol. 2022;18(2):131–8.
49. El-Sayed El-Sayed Gaafar A, Ibrahem Ismail E, Zaghloul HS. Otoacoustic emissions value in patients with idiopathic sudden sensorineural hearing loss. J Otol. 2022;17:183–90.
50. Subirana Pozo FX. Tesis doctoral: productos de distorsión de las otoemisiones acústicas como factor pronóstico de la hipoacusia brusca. Barcelona: Universidad Autónoma de Barcelona; 2021.
51. Wang CT, Huang TW, Kuo SW, Cheng PW. Correlation between audiovestibular function tests and hearing outcomes in severe to profound sudden sensorineural hearing loss. Ear Hear. 2009;30:110–4.
52. Junicho M, Aso S, Fujisaka M, et al. Prognosis of lowtone sudden deafness-does it inevitably progress to Ménière's disease? Acta Otolaryngol. 2008;128:304–8.
53. Fushiki H, Junicho M, Kanazawa Y, et al. Prognosis of sudden low-tone loss other than acute low-tone sensorineural hearing loss. Acta Otolaryngol. 2010;130:559–64.
54. Hornibrook J, Flook E, Greig S, et al. MRI inner ear imaging and tone burst electrocochleography in the diagnosis of Ménière's disease. Otol Neurotol. 2015;36:1109–14.
55. Junicho M, Fushiki H, Aso S, Watanabe Y. Prognostic value of initial electronystagmography findings in idiopathic sudden sensorineural hearing loss without vertigo. Otol Neurotol. 2008;29:905–9.
56. Cho J, Cheon H, Park JH, et al. Sudden sensorineural hearing loss associated with inner ear lesions detected by magnetic resonance imaging. PLoS One. 2017;12:e0186038.

57. Hong SM, Byun JY, Park CH, et al. Saccular damage in patients with idiopathic sudden senso-rineural hearing loss without vertigo. Otolaryngol Head Neck Surg. 2008;139:541–5.
58. Genestar Bosch EI. Tesis doctoral: potenciales evocados vestibulares miogénicos en la sordera brusca. Barcelona: Universidad Autónoma de Barcelona; 2011.
59. Liang M, Wu H, Chen J, et al. Vestibular evoked myogenic potential may predict the hearing recovery in patients with unilateral idiopathic sudden sensorineural hearing loss. Front Neurol. 2022;13:1017608.
60. Niu X, Zhang Y, Zhang Q, et al. The relationship between hearing loss and vestibular dysfunc-tion in patients with sudden sensorineural hearing loss. Acta Otolaryngol. 2016;136:225–31.
61. Pogson JM, Taylor RL, Young AS, et al. Vertigo with sudden hearing loss: audio-vestibular characteristics. J Neurol. 2016;263:2086–96.
62. Battat N, Ungar OJ, Handzel O, et al. Video head impulse test for the assessment of vestibu-lar function of patients with idiopathic sudden sensorineural hearing loss without vertigo. J Laryngol Otol. 2023;137(12):1374–7.
63. Fujimoto C, Egami N, Kinoshita M, et al. Involvement of vestibular organs in idiopathic sudden hearing loss with vertigo: an analysis using oVEMP and cVEMP testing. Clin Neurophysiol. 2015;126:1033–8.
64. Oiticica J, Bittar RS, Castro CC, et al. Contribution of audiovestibular tests to the topographic diagnosis of sudden deafness. Int Arch Otorhinolaryngol. 2013;17:305–14.
65. Lee HS, Song JN, Park JM, et al. Association between vestibular function and hearing out-come in idiopathic sudden sensorineural hearing loss. Korean J Audiol. 2014;18:131–6.
66. Yu H, Li H. Vestibular dysfunctions in sudden sensorineural hearing loss: a systematic review and meta-analysis. Front Neurol. 2018;9:45.
67. Kizkapan DB, Karlidag T, Basar F, et al. Vestibular functions in patients with idiopathic sudden sensorineural hearing loss and its relation to prognosis. Auris Nasus Larynx. 2022;49:374–82.
68. Castellucci A, Botti C, Delmonte S, et al. Vestibular assessment in sudden sensorineural hear-ing loss: role in the prediction of hearing outcome and in the early detection of vascular and hydropic pathomechanisms. Front Neurol. 2023;14:1127008.
69. Hong JP, Lee JY, Kim MB. A comparative study using vestibular mapping in sudden sensorineu-ral hearing loss with and without vertigo. Otolaryngol Head Neck Surg. 2023;169(6):1573–81.
70. Shen J, Ma X, Zhang Q, et al. The functional status of vestibular otolith and conductive path-way in patients with unilateral idiopathic sudden sensorineural hearing loss. Front Neurol. 2023;14:1237516.
71. Hepkarsi S, Kaya I, Kirazli T. Vestibular function assessment in Idiopathic sudden sensori-neural hearing loss: a prospective study. Eur Arch Otorhinolaryngol. 2024;281(5):2365–72.
72. Lin SC, Lin MY. Impact of audiovestibular factors on prognosis in patients with sudden sensori-neural hearing loss without vertigo. Eur Arch Otorhinolaryngol. 2024. https://doi.org/10.1007/s00405-024-08789-5.

MRI in Sudden Sensorineural Hearing Loss

Mayte Herrera, Ana Hernando García,
María Urbasos Pascual, and Guillermo Plaza

Introduction

Once the clinical diagnosis of sudden sensorineural hearing loss (SSNHL) has been established, the healthcare professional considers which imaging study is appropriate to detect possible causes and even a radiological sign with prognostic value regarding hearing improvement [1–5]. At the same time, the reasonable period of time for its performance should also be determined [6].

Magnetic Resonance Imaging in Asymmetric Sensorineural Hearing Loss

Numerous studies have analysed the cost-effectiveness of requesting magnetic resonance imaging (MRI) as a *screening* test for acoustic schwannoma (neurinoma) as its incidence is <2% of total asymmetric hearing loss [7].

For most authors, MRI is indicated if there is an asymmetric sensorineural hearing loss, as Plaza et al. published more than 20 years ago [7], with a difference

M. Herrera (✉)
Ear, Nose and Throat Department, Hospital Universitario de Fuenlabrada, Madrid, Spain

Ear, Nose and Throat Department, Hospital Universitario Sanitas La Zarzuela, Madrid, Spain

A. Hernando García · M. Urbasos Pascual
Diagnostic Imaging Department, Hospital Universitario de Fuenlabrada, Madrid, Spain

G. Plaza
Ear, Nose and Throat Department, Hospital Universitario de Fuenlabrada, Madrid, Spain

Ear, Nose and Throat Department, Hospital Universitario Sanitas La Zarzuela, Madrid, Spain

Universidad Rey Juan Carlos, Madrid, Spain

G. Plaza, J. R. García Berrocal (eds.), *Sudden Sensorineural Hearing Loss*, https://doi.org/10.1007/978-3-031-61385-2_5

Table 1 Protocol for the detection of pathology of the internal auditory canal and pontocerebellar angle

Asymmetric sensorineural hearing loss (interaural PTA difference or speech discrimination threshold >20 dB). Includes SSNHL and rapidly progressive SSNHL
SSNHL associated with neurological symptoms (trigeminal neuralgia, involvement of other cranial nerves, ataxia, etc.)
Unilateral tinnitus with asymmetric hearing loss (still <20 dB). If the tinnitus is pulsatile, MRI indication is also considered, even without hearing loss
Instability and vertigo associated with sensorineural hearing loss <20 dB, even if not asymmetrical
Triad of symptoms of Ménière's disease (vertigo, hearing loss and tinnitus)
Altered AEPs: V-wave latency increase or III-V difference

Taken from Plaza et al. [7]. *AEPs* auditory-evoked potentials

between both ears that is greater than 20 dB [8] or when associated with another symptomatology such as vertigo or tinnitus [9] (Table 1).

There is more discussion about whether a T1-weighted MRI with gadolinium should be performed in all cases or whether a T2-weighted sequence MRI as screening would be sufficient [10]. For some authors, cost-effectiveness studies support the use of T2-weighted MRI [11], but there is no agreement in this regard. In any case, audiological tests are not sufficient, and according to a recent meta-analysis, an imaging test is necessary, even if without contrast [12].

Magnetic Resonance Imaging: Complementary Test of Choice for SSNHL

MRI is the scan of choice for the diagnosis of neurological vascular events such as cerebral ischaemia or haemorrhage, demyelinating diseases or neoplasms, some of which may debut with SSNHL [6].

It is also the benchmark examination for the diagnosis of vestibular schwannoma, where traditionally enhanced sequences are employed in T1-weighted, T2-weighted and 3D-FIESTA/CISS, and may or may not be completed with T1-weighted sequences after gadolinium administration [12].

Currently, there are numerous studies that show the high sensitivity of the 3D-FLAIR sequence, with and without gadolinium contrast, especially in 3 Tesla MRI, to diagnose cochlear alterations, which could be the causes of SSNHL [13–24]. Therefore, at present, in all cases of SSNHL, it is always indicated to perform a cranial MRI and, if possible, within the first month from the onset of the symptoms, to detect cochlear alterations, as recommended in the Spanish consensus [3].

MRI Findings for SSNHL

For many years, it has been evident that there are cases of SSNHL that are related to the existence of a vestibular schwannoma, as it is not uncommon for SSNHL to be the first symptom of the condition [25], so the recommendation to request an MRI in all cases of SSNHL was established to rule out vestibular schwannoma, as it could be the symptom of the onset of the tumour. This indication should be maintained, even if there is recovery of hearing spontaneously or with treatment [26–31].

At the end of the twentieth century, several series of vestibular schwannomas were presented, analysing how many had a history of SSNHL (Table 2). In a recent review from Japan on 686 patients diagnosed with vestibular schwannoma, 232 (33.81%) had suffered from SSNHL at some point in their evolution (not only at onset), unrelated to tumour size. Of the 172 cases analysed, 119 had a single episode of SSNHL, but 44 (6.41%) had two episodes. With steroid treatment, hearing recovery was obtained in 61% of the first episodes and in 45% of the second episodes, that is, the hearing improvement of SSNHL does not rule out that there may be a vestibular schwannoma [32]. However, in a retrospective series from China on 1383 patients with vestibular schwannoma, only 10 cases initially presented with SSNHL (0.7%) [33].

From another perspective, the key question is about the likelihood of having a vestibular schwannoma if a patient suffers from SSNHL (Fig. 1). In 1995, Weber et al. [34] published a study with 16 patients diagnosed with SSNHL who underwent an MRI, observing in one case a lesion of multiple sclerosis, another with a meningioma of the pontocerebellar angle and a third with a vestibular schwannoma. They concluded that MRI is an essential examination in the study and management of SSNHL, as in their case series it determines the cause of SSNHL up to 18.75%. Also in 1995, Saunders et al. [35] reported a series of 837 cases of SSNHL, in which

Table 2 Incidence of SSNHL in patients with vestibular schwannoma

Author (year)	Vestibular schwannoma	Patients diagnosed with SSNHL	Percentage
Edwards et al. (1951)	157	5	3.2%
Higgs (1973)	44	4	9.1%
Kusakari et al. (1979)	54	2	3.7%
Yosimito et al. (1981)	78	5	6.4%
Pensak et al. (1985)	498	69	13.9%
Berg et al. (1986)	133	17	12.8%
Komatsuzaki et al. (1987)	100	11	11%
Ogawa et al. (1991)	132	–	22%
Yanaginara et al. (1993)	111	–	28%
Aslan et al. (1997)	192	14	–
Takahashi et al. (2022)	686	232	33.8%
Song et al. (2022)	1383	10	0.7%

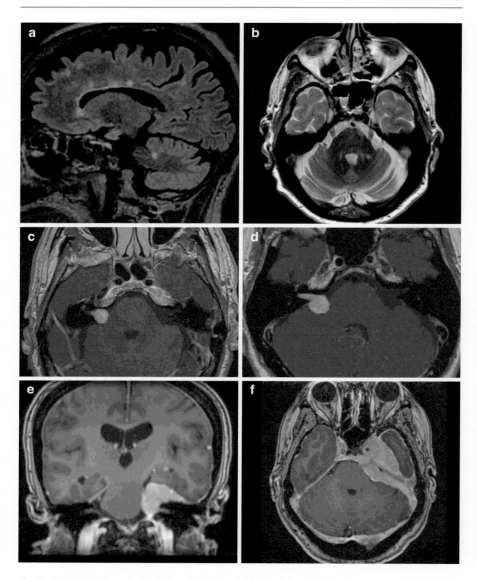

Fig. 1 (**a, b**) FLAIR sagittal MRI and FSET2 axial MRI with multiple white matter demyelinating lesions compatible with multiple sclerosis, with protuberant involvement and left middle cerebellar peduncle. (**c, d**) SET1 axial MRI with gadolinium (several cases) showing a right intracanalicular enhanced tumour compatible with neurinoma of the eighth cranial nerve, with cisternal component. (**e, f**) T1-weighted axial and coronal MRI with GD showing extensive left pontocerebellar meningioma with canalicular extension, also affecting the cavernous sinus and the homolateral middle cranial fossa

MRI was able to diagnose 13 vestibular schwannomas, an incidence of 2.5%. Like other authors, they recommend conducting an MRI with gadolinium in all cases of SSNHL.

In 2004, Aarnisalo et al. [36] published a review of 82 patients with SSNHL who underwent an MRI, finding pathology in 35% of cases, although this was the cause of SSNHL in only 7% of cases: four vestibular schwannomas (5%), an internal carotid artery obstruction (1%) and a cerebral infarction (1%). They reported that up to 10% of vestibular schwannomas and 7% of patients with Ménière's disease debut with SSNHL as an onset symptom. They concluded that an MRI should be performed in less than 14 days from the diagnosis of SSNHL as other aetiologies should be excluded to consider it idiopathic.

More recently, Fujita et al. [37] found a 3% incidence of vestibular schwannoma in a series of 499 SSNHL cases, while a meta-analysis by the US Congress of Neurological Surgeons estimated it at 2.8%. In any case, this was well above the incidence in the normal population, which is estimated at 0.02%. Yang et al. [38] reviewed 1249 patients diagnosed with SSNHL, finding an incidence of vestibular schwannoma of only 1.12% (14 cases). Lee et al. [28] reviewed 1698 cases of SSNHL, of which 43 patients (2.53%) had vestibular schwannoma. Of these, 11 cases (34%) had a good response to steroid treatment, stating again that hearing improvement in SSNHL does not rule out the possibility of a vestibular schwannoma [27].

MRI Cochlear Findings in Idiopathic Sudden Sensorineural Hearing Loss (ISSNHL)

In addition to the screening of possible causes of SSNHL, MRI allows us to study the anatomy and pathology of the inner ear in an excellent way through 3D reconstructions, leading to a topographic and physiopathology study of each case, as magnificently illustrated in several series and reviews [13–24, 39, 40] (Fig. 2).

These studies currently show the high sensitivity of the 3D-FLAIR sequence, before and after gadolinium administration, to identify alterations in the inner ear signal, such as labyrinthitis or cochlear haemorrhage, which could go unnoticed or be recognised later in the traditional T1-weighted and T2-weighted sequences [6, 13, 21, 24].

In ISSNHL, an increase in the FLAIR sequence signal in the affected labyrinth suggests a small haemorrhage within it or a higher protein concentration due to an increase in its permeability. In addition, the presence of enhancement in the inner ear after gadolinium injection is considered a sign of rupture of the blood labyrinth barrier (BLB) [13, 21, 24]. In other words, under normal conditions no baseline hypersignal is observed in the inner ear in the 3D-FLAIR sequence or post-contrast reinforcement. Therefore, the presence of these findings suggests certain involvement of the inner ear in relation to ISSNHL.

In 2006, Sugiura et al. [15] published the first article referring to the use of the 3D-FLAIR sequence for the study of ISSNHL. In a sample of eight patients, 50%

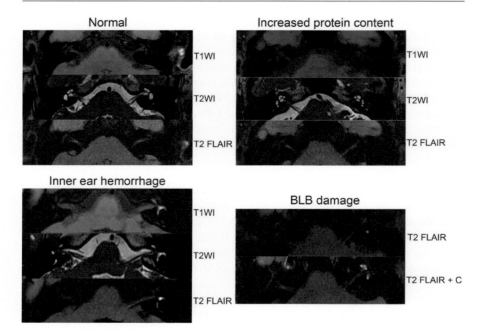

Fig. 2 Representative 3D-FLAIR MRI images of different groups. The images of normal patients (top left) show that the structure of the bilateral inner ear was symmetrical, and the morphology and signal of the bilateral cochlea, vestibule and semicircular canal were normal. The images of patients with protein deposition (top right) show that the structure of the bilateral inner ear was also symmetrical. There was a slightly higher signal of T2-FLAIR in the right cochlea. The T2WI signal increased significantly only in the right cochlea. The images of the inner haemorrhage (bottom left) show that the T2-FLAIR signal increased in the right cochlea, vestibule and semicircular canal. The intensity of both T1WI and T2WI signals increased. The images of the BLB damage (bottom left) show that the T2-FLAIR signal increased in the right cochlea. The signal intensity of T1WI did not increase. The intensity of the T2WI signal increased. After the enhancement of the scan, the signal of the right cochlea was slightly enhanced. (Reprinted with permission from: Wang M, Hu N, Wang Y, et al. Clinical value of 3D-FLAIR MRI in idiopathic sudden sensorineural hearing loss. ACS Chem Neurosci. 2022; 13: 151–7. Copyright (2022) American Chemical Society [21])

showed a cochlear pathological signal, and it could be assumed that the pathology causing their sudden hearing loss was in the inner ear. Likewise, if associated vertigo existed, there was also a hypersignal in the vestibule. This article considers for the first time the possibility of using MRI as a prognostic method in the follow-up of patients with positive findings in the cochlear FLAIR image.

Along the same lines, in 2008, Yoshida et al. [16] published a study of 48 patients with ISSNHL evaluated by MRI with baseline 3D-FLAIR sequence, suggesting that patients with hypersignal in FLAIR in the affected ear have a worse prognosis, which is reflected in a poor final hearing gain of this group compared to the group that did not show signal alterations.

In 2013, Berrettini et al. [13] performed an analysis of the use of the 3D-FLAIR sequence in patients with ISSNHL. They performed 3 T MRI with FIESTA

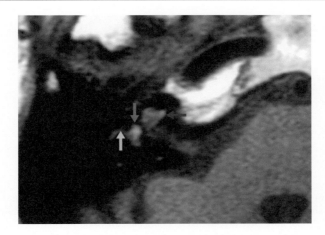

Fig. 3 MRI in T1-weighted sequence without contrast: haemorrhagic pattern. Hyperintense signal in the cochlea and vestibule and part of the lateral semicircular canal (blue arrows). (Plontke SK. Diagnostics and therapy of sudden hearing loss. GMS Curr Top Otorhinolaryngol Head Neck Surg. 2018 Feb 19;16:Doc05. doi: 10.3205/cto000144 [39] (https://creativecommons.org/licenses/by/4.0/))

sequences, 3D-FLAIR and T1-weighted FSE (both pre- and post-gadolinium). Out of a sample size of 23 patients, 57% showed positive MRI findings with three possible radiological patterns:

1. Pattern 1: Haemorrhagic pattern (cochlear haemorrhage). High signal in T1 due to subacute methaemoglobin and high signal in FLAIR due to increased protein content in endo- and perilymphatic fluid secondary to the presence of methaemoglobin (Fig. 3).
2. Pattern 2: Inflammatory pattern. High signal in FLAIR due to exudative increase in protein content in endo- and perilymphatic fluid. There are no alterations in T1 (Fig. 4).
3. Pattern 3: Rupture of the blood–labyrinth barrier (BLB). Enhancement after gadolinium injection secondary to BLB rupture, usually more evident in the FLAIR sequence than in T1. This can be associated with both patterns 1 and 2.

Thus, when hypersignal is observed in FLAIR sequence, it can be assumed that there is a change in the protein composition of the inner ear, which may be due to a haemorrhagic component or an acute inflammatory process. Findings can also be observed that translate rupture of the BLB as neural enhancement or in endo/perilymphatic fluid following gadolinium injection. In fact, the 3D-FLAIR sequence is more sensitive than the T1-weighted sequence to identify enhancements due to rupture of the BLB and small intralabyrinthine haemorrhagic alterations, and improves its accuracy when performed with fat suppression [6].

In their study, Berrettini et al. [13] concluded that MRI with 3D-FLAIR sequence increases diagnostic sensitivity by 50%. Patients with positive MRI findings showed

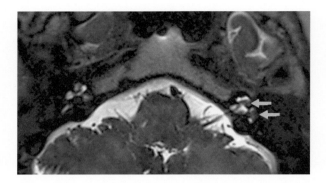

Fig. 4 MRI in T2-weighted sequence: inflammatory pattern (no hypersignal in T1-weighted). Hyperintense signal in the cochlea and vestibule and part of the lateral semicircular canal. (Taken from Plontke (2017). https://creativecommons.org/licenses/by/4.0/. Plontke SK. Diagnostics and therapy of sudden hearing loss. GMS Curr Top Otorhinolaryngol Head Neck Surg. 2018 Feb 19;16:Doc05. doi: 10.3205/cto000144 [39])

a greater presence of vertigo and worse previous PTA as statistically significant data. However, there was no difference in the final recovery. The average number of days to perform the MRI was 12. And 46% of the positives had only one affection site.

Similarly, Lee et al. [17] studied the usefulness of MRI with 3D-FLAIR as a prognostic value. Out of 120 patients, those with positive findings in 3D-FLAIR sequence (25.8%) were distinguished from non-positive patients, with a significant difference in the final PTA between the two groups. It can therefore be concluded that patients without MRI signal alterations in the inner ear have a better prognosis.

Several meta-analyses confirm the importance of 3D-FLAIR MRI for ISSNHL [18–20]. The presence of a high signal in the MRI indicates more severe ISSNHL, is associated with vertigo (OR 2.88) and correlates with a lower rate of hearing improvement, so its early performance for ISSNHL is recommended to help determine its prognosis.

Vivas et al. [41] reported a series of 11 cases of ISSNHL with diagnosis of labyrinthine MR haemorrhage in 3D-FLAIR sequence, confirming that it is a marker of a poor prognosis of ISSNHL, with an auditory response in less than 20% of patients. Wang et al. [21] analysed 1300 cases of SSNHL with 3D-FLAIR MRI, demonstrating that it was normal in 739 cases; that there was cochlear haemorrhage in 218, that there was an inflammatory pattern with exudative increase in protein content in 288 cases and that there were signs of BLB rupture in 55 cases, confirming greater severity if there was cochlear haemorrhage. Compagnone et al. [22] presented 36 cases of SSNHL in which MRI in 3D-FLAIR sequence defined enhancement at the base of the cochlea in all cases, but apical only in 73% and vestibular in 50%. When there was vestibular enhancement, the prognosis was worse. Conte et al. [24] reviewed 50 cases of ISSNHL that underwent an MRI in the first 72 h after diagnosis, finding alterations in 80% of severe cases, but not in mild ones, and with a worse prognosis and higher relapse rate.

In Spain, there have been some publications of cases of ISSNHL with cochlear alterations in MRI [42, 43]. At the Hospital Puerta de Hierro in Majadahonda (Madrid), a protocol has been implemented to perform the MRI early with the intention of increasing the possibility of these diagnoses (Fig. 5).

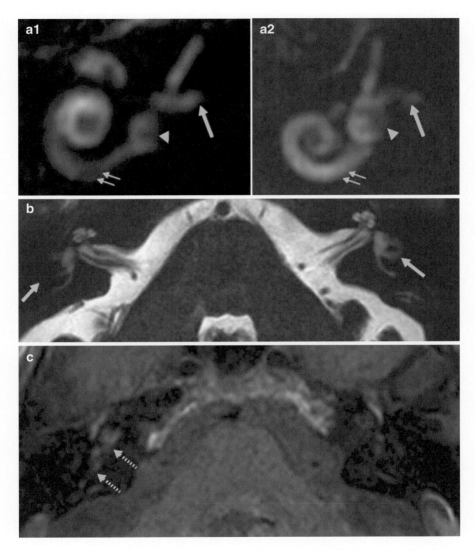

Fig. 5 MRI in an ISSNHL case associated with anticoagulants. (**a1**) T2-weighted sequence, DRIVE, right sagittal reconstruction. (**a2**) T2-weighted sequence, DRIVE, left sagittal reconstruction. (**b**) T2-weighted sequence, axial. Signal defects are observed in the basal cochlea (*double arrow*), vestibule (*arrowhead*) and lateral semicircular canal, compared to the normal left side. (**c**) T1-weighted sequence, axial. A spontaneous hypersignal is observed in the inner ear, haemorrhagic pattern (*dashed arrow*). (Courtesy of Beatriz Arellano and Beatriz Brea, Puerta de Hierro University Hospital, Majadahonda)

Therefore, MRI would currently have two uses for SSNHL: on the one hand, for an aetiological diagnosis; on the other, for the detection of signs with potential prognostic value. With MRI, moreover, we are able to endorse the vascular theory of ISSNHL, given that there are numerous articles in the literature of cases of bleeding in the inner ear as a cause of sudden sensorineural hearing loss. All of them emphasise that patients with pathological hypersignal in MRI have more vestibular symptoms and a worse auditory prognosis. However, in patients with mild hearing loss, there is no pathological hypersignal in the cochlea in the MRI.

In 2017, Conte et al. [23] studied the effect that performing an early MRI with 3D-FLAIR sequence could have on treatment and, therefore, on the prognosis of SSNHL, as several meta-analyses have later confirmed [17–20]. These authors recommend the following protocol for performing MRI for SSNHL:

1. With a 3 Tesla MRI scanner, thanks to its greater resolution.
2. High-resolution 3D-FIESTA (CISS) axial sequence, allowing clear visualisation of the entire cisternal neural pathway.
3. Baseline and post-contrast T1-weighted FSE sequence. Identification of subacute cochlear haemorrhages and small vestibular schwannomas.
4. Baseline and post-contrast 3D-FLAIR sequence. Early identification of small intralabyrinthine haemorrhages and signs of BLB rupture.

Furthermore, Kurata et al. [44] recently presented a series of 287 cases of acute sensorineural hearing loss, finding that the detection rates of abnormal MRI findings vary significantly. A hyperintense signal on delayed 3D-FLAIR was observed in all patients with intralabyrinthine schwannoma or vestibular schwannoma and 20.5% of patients with ISSNHL but was rarely observed in definite Ménière's disease (MD, 2.6%). In contrast, endolymphatic hydrops (EH) was frequently observed in patients with definite MD (79.5%) but was observed much less frequently in patients with ISSNHL (11.0%). Similarly, Seo et al. [45] and Cai et al. [46] reported that those cases evolving from ISSNHL to a definite MD have more commonly EH, low-tone descending hearing loss and vertigo after a multifactor regression analysis.

Conclusions

MRI is indicated in all cases of SSNHL, even if there has been improvement with corticosteroid treatment. It should be performed within the first month from the start of symptoms as soon as possible. The purpose of the MRI is to recognise causal lesions and possible alterations of the cochlear or vestibular signal that could have a prognostic value. Baseline and post-contrast 3D-FLAIR sequences with gadolinium increase MRI sensitivity in SSNHL imaging. Prospective studies are needed that can assess the correlation of MRI findings with treatment effectiveness and decide whether it may be useful in the follow-up of ISSNHL.

References

1. Rauch SD. Clinical practice. Idiopathic sudden sensorineural hearing loss. N Engl J Med. 2008;359:833–40.
2. Plaza G, Durio E, Herráiz C, Asociación Madrileña de ORL, et al. Consenso sobre el diagnóstico y tratamiento de la sordera súbita. Acta Otorrinolaringol Esp. 2011;62:144–57.
3. Herrera M, García Berrocal JR, García Arumí A, et al. Update on consensus on diagnosis and treatment of idiopathic sudden sensorineural hearing loss. Acta Otorrinolaringol Esp (Engl Ed). 2019;70:290–300.
4. Stachler RJ, Chandrasekhar SS, Archer SM, American Academy of Otolaryngology-Head and Neck Surgery, et al. Clinical practice guideline: sudden hearing loss. Otolaryngol Head Neck Surg. 2012;146(3 Suppl):S1–35.
5. Chandrasekhar SS, Tsai Do BS, Schwartz SR, et al. Clinical practice guideline: sudden hearing loss (update). Otolaryngol Head Neck Surg. 2019;161(Suppl. 1):S1–S45.
6. Herrera Mera M, Hernando García A, Ramos López M, et al. Diagnóstico por la imagen en la sordera súbita. In: Plaza G, editor. Sordera súbita: diagnóstico y tratamiento. Madrid: Ergon; 2018. p. 127–37.
7. Plaza G, López Lafuente J, Aparicio JM, et al. Resonancia magnética: prueba de elección en el despistaje de tumores del conducto auditivo interno y ángulo pontocerebeloso. Acta Otorrinolaringol Esp. 2001;52:651–6.
8. Gupta A, Monsell EM. Which patients with asymmetric sensorineural hearing loss should undergo imaging? Laryngoscope. 2018;128:1990–1.
9. Ahsan SF, Standring R, Osborn DA, et al. Clinical predictors of abnormal magnetic resonance imaging findings in patients with asymmetric sensorineural hearing loss. JAMA Otolaryngol Head Neck Surg. 2015;141:451–6.
10. Hentschel M, Scholte M, Steens S, et al. The diagnostic accuracy of non-imaging screening protocols for vestibular schwannoma in patients with asymmetrical hearing loss and/or unilateral audiovestibular dysfunction: a diagnostic review and meta-analysis. Clin Otolaryngol. 2017;42:815–23.
11. Coelho DH, Tang Y, Suddarth B, et al. MRI surveillance of vestibular schwannomas without contrast enhancement: clinical and economic evaluation. Laryngoscope. 2018;128:202–9.
12. Hentschel MA, Kunst HPM, Rovers MM, et al. Diagnostic accuracy of high-resolution T2-weighted MRI vs contrast-enhanced T1-weighted MRI to screen for cerebellopontine angle lesions in symptomatic patients. Clin Otolaryngol. 2018;43:805–11.
13. Berrettini S, Seccia V, Fortunato S, et al. Analysis of the 3-dimensional fluid-attenuated inversion-recovery (3D-FLAIR) sequence in idiopathic sudden sensorineural hearing loss. JAMA Otolaryngol Head Neck Surg. 2013;139:456–64.
14. Lee HY, Jung SY, Park MS, et al. Feasibility of three-dimensional fluid-attenuated inversion recovery magnetic resonance imaging as a prognostic factor in patients with sudden hearing loss. Eur Arch Otorrinolaringol. 2012;269:1885–91.
15. Sugiura M, Naganawa S, Teranishi M, et al. Three-dimensional fluid-attenuated inversion recovery magnetic resonance imaging findings in patients with sudden sensorineural hearing loss. Laryngoscope. 2006;116:1451–4.
16. Yoshida T, Sugiura M, Naganawa S, et al. Three-dimensional fluid-attenuated inversion recovery magnetic resonance imaging findings and prognosis in sudden sensorineural hearing loss. Laryngoscope. 2008;118:1433–7.
17. Lee JI, Yoon RG, Lee JH, et al. Prognostic value of labyrinthine 3D-FLAIR abnormalities in idiopathic sudden sensorineural hearing loss. AJNR Am J Neuroradiol. 2016;37:2317–22.
18. Gao Z, Chi FL. The clinical value of three-dimensional fluid-attenuated inversion recovery magnetic resonance imaging in patients with idiopathic sudden sensorineural hearing loss: a meta-analysis. Otol Neurotol. 2014;35:1730–5.

19. Lammers MJW, Young E, Fenton D, et al. The prognostic value and pathophysiologic significance of three-dimensional fluid-attenuated inversion recovery (3D-FLAIR) magnetic resonance imaging in idiopathic sudden sensorineural hearing loss: a systematic review and meta-analysis. Clin Otolaryngol. 2019;44:1017–25.
20. Yoon RG, Choi Y, Park HJ. Clinical usefulness of labyrinthine three-dimensional fluid-attenuated inversion recovery magnetic resonance images in idiopathic sudden sensorineural hearing loss. Curr Opin Otolaryngol Head Neck Surg. 2021;29:349–56.
21. Wang M, Hu N, Wang Y, et al. Clinical value of 3D-FLAIR MRI in idiopathic sudden sensorineural hearing loss. ACS Chem Neurosci. 2022;13:151–7.
22. Compagnone L, Levigne V, Pereira B, et al. Injected 3T-3D-FLAIR-MRI labyrinthine patterns match with the severity and tonotopic alteration in sudden sensorineural hearing loss. Eur Arch Otorrinolaringol. 2022;279:4883–91.
23. Conte G, Di Berardino F, Sina C, et al. MR imaging in sudden sensorineural hearing loss. Time to talk. AJNR Am J Neuroradiol. 2017;38:1475–9.
24. Conte G, Di Berardino F, Mastrapasqua RF, et al. Prognostic value of early magnetic resonance imaging patterns in sudden hearing loss. Audiol Neurootol. 2022;27:64–74.
25. Chaimoff M, Nageris BI, Sulkes J, et al. Sudden hearing loss as a presenting symptom of acoustic neuroma. Am J Otolaryngol. 1999;20:157–60.
26. Berenholz LP, Eriksen C, Hirsh FA. Recovery from repeated sudden hearing loss with corticosteroid use in the presence of an acoustic neuroma. Ann Otol Rhinol Laryngol. 1992;101:827–31.
27. Puccinelli C, Carlson ML. Improvement or recovery from sudden sensorineural hearing loss with steroid therapy does not preclude the need for MRI to rule out vestibular schwannoma. Otol Neurotol. 2019;40:674–80.
28. Lee SA, Kim SY, Lee Y, Lee JD. Efficacy of steroid treatment for sudden sensorineural hearing loss in patients with vestibular schwannoma. Acta Otolaryngol. 2022;142:402–5.
29. Nakamura Y, Kurioka T, Sano H, et al. Clinical characteristics and corticosteroid responses of acoustic neuroma treated as idiopathic sudden sensorineural hearing loss. J Int Adv Otol. 2023;19:5–9.
30. Shilo S, Hannaux O, Gilboa D, et al. Could the audiometric criteria for sudden sensorineural hearing loss miss vestibular schwannomas? Laryngoscope. 2023;133:670–5.
31. Huynh PP, Saba ES, Hoerter JE, Jiang N. Steroid efficacy on audiologic recovery in patients with sudden sensorineural hearing loss and vestibular schwannoma: a retrospective review. Otol Neurotol. 2023;44:780–5.
32. Takahashi M, Inagaki A, Aihara N, et al. Acoustic neuromas associated with sudden sensorineural hearing loss. Acta Otolaryngol. 2022;142:415–8.
33. Song M, Wang D, Li J, et al. Sudden sensorineural hearing loss as the initial symptom in patients with acoustic neuroma. Front Neurol. 2022;13:953265.
34. Weber PC, Zbar RI, Gantz BJ. Appropriateness of magnetic resonance imaging in sudden sensorineural hearing loss. Otolaryngol Head Neck Surg. 1997;116:153–6.
35. Saunders JE, Luxford WM, Devgan KK, et al. Sudden hearing loss in acoustic neuroma patients. Otolaryngol Head Neck Surg. 1995;113:23–31.
36. Aarnisalo AA, Suoranta H, Ylikoski J. Magnetic resonance imaging findings in the auditory pathway of patients with sudden deafness. Otol Neurotol. 2004;25:245–9.
37. Fujita T, Saito K, Kashiwagi N, et al. The prevalence of vestibular schwannoma among patients treated as sudden sensorineural hearing loss. Auris Nasus Larynx. 2019;46:78–82.
38. Yang W, Mei X, Li X, et al. The prevalence and clinical characteristics of vestibular schwannoma among patients treated as sudden sensorineural hearing loss: a 10-year retrospective study in southern China. Am J Otolaryngol. 2020;41:102452.
39. Plontke SK. Diagnostics and therapy of sudden hearing loss. GMS Curr Top Otorhinolaryngol Head Neck Surg. 2018;16:Doc05. https://doi.org/10.3205/cto000144.
40. Araújo-Martins J, Melo P, Ribeiro C, Barros E. Recovery of cochlear and vestibular function after labyrinthine haemorrhage. Acta Medica Port. 2014;27:649–51.

41. Vivas EX, Panella NJ, Baugnon KL. Spontaneous labyrinthine hemorrhage: a case series. Otolaryngol Head Neck Surg. 2018;159:908–13.
42. Avilés Jurado FJ, Salvadó E, Domènech E, et al. Hemorragia intralaberíntica. Acta Otorrinolaringol Esp. 2010;61:465–7.
43. Herrero Agustín J, González Martín FM, Pinilla Urraca M, et al. Hemorragia coclear. Causa excepcional de sordera súbita sensorineural. Acta Otorrinolaringol Esp. 2002;53:363–8.
44. Kurata N, Kawashima Y, Ito T, et al. Advanced magnetic resonance imaging sheds light on the distinct pathophysiology of various types of acute sensorineural hearing loss. Otol Neurotol. 2023;44(7):656–63.
45. Seo HW, Kim Y, Kim HJ, et al. Findings of intravenous gadolinium inner ear MRI in patients with acute low-tone sensorineural hearing loss. Clin Exp Otorhinolaryngol. 2023;16(4):334–41.
46. Cai H, Xiao H, Lin J, et al. The value of gadolinium-enhanced MRI in predicting the development of sudden hearing loss into Ménière's disease. Clin Otolaryngol. 2024;49(1):117–23.

Prognostic Factors and Recovery Criteria in Sudden Sensorineural Hearing Loss

Carlos O'Connor-Reina, Laura Rodríguez-Alcalá,
Felipe Benjumea Flores, Juan Carlos Casado Morente,
and Guillermo Plaza

Introduction

Sudden sensorineural hearing loss (SSNHL) is a sudden decrease or loss of hearing defined in audiometric criteria based on severity and the course of time. Fortunately, most cases are unilateral [1–6].

The distribution between sexes seems to be almost equal. It affects people of all age groups, with a maximum incidence between 30 and 60 years of age.

Before mentioning the different prognostic factors involved in idiopathic SSNHL (ISSNHL), we should take into account that this condition presents a spontaneous recovery in up to 35–60% of affected patients and with thresholds of up to 35–40 dB [6–10]. A recent meta-analysis on spontaneous recovery of ISSNHL including 13 articles showed a pooled spontaneous recovery of 60.28% (95% confidence interval [CI] = 38.88–79.94%) with a heterogeneity of 86.0% (95% CI = 69.4–93.6%) [11]. This very high spontaneous rate is a lot difficult to determine the actual prognosis of the disease and evaluate its possible treatments.

Many prognostic factors for ISSNHL have been described: age, severity of hearing loss and audiometric curve, delayed treatment, tinnitus, vertigo and cardiovascular risk factors [3, 5, 6]. Therefore, it has been shown that the most severe initial hearing loss, advanced age, the presence of vertigo, a descending-type audiogram,

C. O'Connor-Reina (✉) · L. Rodríguez-Alcalá · F. Benjumea Flores · J. C. Casado Morente
Ear, Nose and Throat Department, Hospitales Quirónsalud Marbella and Campo de Gibraltar, Cádiz, Spain
e-mail: coconnor@us.es

G. Plaza
Ear, Nose and Throat Department, Hospital Universitario de Fuenlabrada, Madrid, Spain

Ear, Nose and Throat Department, Hospital Universitario Sanitas La Zarzuela, Madrid, Spain

Universidad Rey Juan Carlos, Madrid, Spain

© The Author(s), under exclusive license to Springer Nature Switzerland AG 2024
G. Plaza, J. R. García Berrocal (eds.), *Sudden Sensorineural Hearing Loss*,
https://doi.org/10.1007/978-3-031-61385-2_6

cardiovascular risk factors such as diabetes, hypercholesterolaemia and hyperglycaemia correlate negatively with hearing recovery in most cases [12–14].

Severity of Hearing Loss

In patients with SSNHL, 10–35% suffer severe or profound sensorineural hearing loss (>80 dB). These patients have a poor prognosis, whereby persistent severe hearing loss seriously affects their quality of life. Despite efforts to clarify its pathophysiological characteristics, the cause of profound SSNHL is still unclear. In such patients, the possibility of spontaneous recovery is more remote [6, 7]. In fact, the prognosis of profound SSNHL is very poor, especially if presented with vertigo and cardiovascular risk factors [12–14].

Recent research such as that of Wei et al. [12] has shown that inner ear haemorrhage is one of the leading causes of profound SSNHL. In their study, out of 80 cases, patients with inner ear haemorrhage accounted for 37.5% of patients with profound ISSNHL; a high incidence compared to other case series where the previously reported incidence of inner ear haemorrhage was 18.6%. This difference may be due to the fact that not all patients with profound ISSNHL underwent magnetic resonance imaging (MRI) of the inner ear (Fig. 1).

In addition, MRI technology has improved in recent years (RM-3T and T2W-3D-FLAIR sequences), making it possible for MRIs to detect inner ear haemorrhage more frequently [15]. The clinical characteristics of these patients were profound hearing loss and vestibular dysfunction. These results support the assumption that their symptoms were caused by inner ear haemorrhage, leading to a worse prognosis [16, 17], as shown by Wang et al. [18], Compagnone et al. [19] and Cointe et al. [20] (see chapter "MRI in Sudden Sensorineural Hearing").

As for patients without inner ear haemorrhage, the main aetiology of profound SSNHL may be related to labyrinthine infarction. Depending on the supply pattern of the cochlea and vestibule, if the infarction only affects the artery that supplies the vestibule, vestibular symptoms may develop first, and when the infarction progresses and affects the supply artery of the cochlea, cochlear symptoms will appear. If the artery supplying the cochlea is affected at an early stage, only cochlear symptoms appear at onset, while vestibular symptoms develop only after the infarction

Fig. 1 Example of inner ear haemorrhage shown by magnetic resonance imaging. The white arrows indicate a high signal strength in T1WI (**a**) and 3D-FLAIR (**b**)

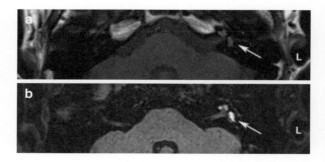

progresses and/or affects the artery supplying the vestibule. Finally, if the infarction lesion is extensive and affects the common trunk of the labyrinthine artery, dual cochlear and vestibular symptoms will be present at onset, resulting in full-frequency hearing loss associated with severe vertigo [6].

Prognostic Factors in ISSNHL

Mattox et al. [7, 21] proposed an ISSNHL staging system, similar to TNM for tumours, which, however, has not come into widespread use (Table 1). This system used the acronym HEAR (*Hearing* for severity of hearing loss; *Elapsed* time up to initial treatment; *Audiogram* shape and *Related* vestibular symptoms). Thus, a patient treated in the first week for ISSNHL with a PTA of 35 dB, an ascending curve and no vertigo would be a H35E1A0R0; meanwhile, another patient who attends an appointment 4 weeks after onset, with a PTA of 80 dB, descending curve and intense vertigo, would be a H80E4R2.

Cvorovic et al. [22] performed a multivariate analysis where the most important factors for the prognosis of ISSNHL were the severity of hearing loss, presence of vertigo, time between onset and treatment, hearing of the other ear and shape of the audiogram. With these, they developed the following recovery (R) prediction formula: (β coefficient was −0.216, −0.231, 0.211, 0.113, and 0.064; the constant, 0.968):

$$R = 0.968 - 0.216 \times S - 0.231 \times V + 0.211 \times T + 0.113 \times OE - 0.064\,A$$

where S indicates severity, V indicates vertigo, T indicates onset time, OE indicates other ear and A indicates audiogram shape.

This R-value was transformed into a probability percentage of hearing improvement values. Thus, for example, a patient with a 40–60 dB hearing loss, without associated vertigo, with good contralateral hearing and who started treatment in the first 4 days, has a probability of improvement of 80% (Fig. 2, blue circle); meanwhile, if the hearing loss is 60–80 dB, with associated vertigo, with affected contralateral ear and late treatment, this probability of improvement decreases to 30% (Fig. 2, red circle).

Table 1 Staging of ISSNHL using the acronym HEAR (modified from Mattox and Lyles [21])

H	*Hearing loss*	Hearing loss PTA: 500, 1000, 2000 Hz
E	*Elapsed time since onset*	Elapsed time since onset (weeks)
A	*Audiogram shape*	Audiogram shape 0. Flat, central or upward sloping 1. Downward sloping
R	*Related vestibular symptoms*	Related vestibular symptoms 0. None 1. Minor 2. Severe or limiting

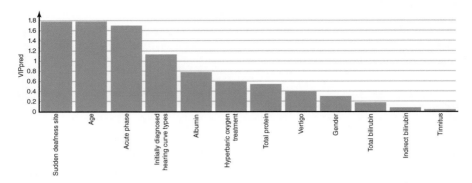

Fig. 2 Severity of hearing loss significantly related to site, age, acute phase, curve type and albumin. (Taken from Lin W, Xiong G, Yan K, et al. Clinical features and influencing factors for the prognosis of patients with sudden deafness. Front Neurol. 2022;13:905069 [22] (https://creativecommons.org/licenses/by/4.0/))

Bing et al. [23], based on a database of 1220 patients in China, using *big data* methodology, concluded that delayed treatment and the initial severity of ISSNHL are the most relevant factors. Similarly, Shimanuki et al. [24], in a sample of 332 patients, found that the prognosis of ISSNHL is related to age, baseline hearing levels, delay time from onset to treatment, diabetes, hypertension and the presence of vertigo. As a post-treatment prognostic factor, they concluded that, if there is no hearing improvement of ≥ 10 dB on days 6–7 after treatment initiation, hearing is unlikely to recover.

Other recent case series reinforce that the most relevant prognostic factors are age, type of audiometric curve and delayed treatment [12–14, 25–29]. Lin et al. [25] reviewed 500 patients with ISSNHL from China and found that age, type of hearing curve at the initial diagnosis, acute phase and sudden deafness site were found to be independently associated with the prognoses of patients with sudden deafness. Through orthogonal partial least-squares discriminant analysis, the sudden deafness site was found to be an indicator with the highest predictive power (Fig. 2).

Lee et al. [26], using artificial intelligence, reviewed the medical data of 453 patients with ISSNHL, showing that the initial audiogram shape is the most important prognostic factor (Fig. 3). Zhou et al. [27] and Wu et al. [28] have proposed normograms for early prediction of ISSNHL prognosis. Once again, hearing loss type, duration from onset to treatment and vertigo are closely associated with hearing recovery. Artificial intelligence, machine learning and deep neural network models are generating algorithms to determine the prognosis of each patient with ISSNH, as reviewed by Aghakhani et al. [29], Uhm et al. [30] and Huang et al. [31].

However, of these prognostic factors, the only one that we can improve is the delay to start treatment by accelerating the diagnostic process [6, 32–38]. For most authors, treatment is considered to be more effective if initiated within the

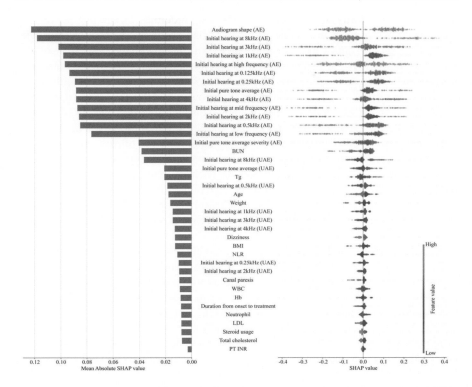

Fig. 3 The feature importance of each prognostic factor appears in each bar plot and the SHAP summary plot. The left bar plot represents the importance of the variables with their overall contribution to the model prediction. The right dot plot represents the directionality with the contribution of the individual values for each variable. The red colour indicates larger values, while the blue colour indicates lower values for each variable. *SHAP* SHapley Additive exPlanation, *AE* affected ear, *BUN* blood urea nitrogen, *UAE* unaffected ear, *Tg* triglyceride, *BMI* body mass index, *NLR* neutrophil–lymphocyte ratio, *WBC* white blood cell, *Hb* haemoglobin, *LDL* low-density lipoprotein, *PT* prothrombin time, *INR* international normalised ratio. (https://creativecommons.org/licenses/by/4.0/. Taken from Lee MK, Jeon ET, Baek N, et al. Prediction of hearing recovery in unilateral sudden sensorineural hearing loss using artificial intelligence. Sci Rep. 2022;12:3977 [23])

first 7 days. A recent meta-analysis has clearly shown that unilateral ISSNHL should be considered a medical emergency because initiating treatment before 3 days have elapsed since the event portends the best outcome: an odds ratio (OR) of 0.42 (95% confidence interval [CI], 0.25–0.71) favouring early treatment was found [35]. Unfortunately, other patients whose treatment starts very late, even after 30 days from onset, have a much worse prognosis, with recovery rates of <25% [6, 36].

Although not always recommended in clinical guidelines, laboratory exams may allow the ENT to have predictors of good or bad prognosis to each patient with ISSNHL. Several studies have shown that serum fibrinogen and several cytokines are good biomarkers for ISSNHL prognosis. Kanzaki et al. [37] showed that high fibrinogen levels measured within 7 days after ISSNHL onset correlated with poorer hearing recovery. Similarly, Okuda el al [38]. showed that the prognosis was significantly better in patients with low fibrinogen levels and high IL-1β levels. Oya et al. [39] presented a meta-analysis including 19 articles, although only 2 included the fibrinogen level with recovery rates showing again that the fibrinogen level of the recovery group was lower than that of the no recovery group. Many other studies have evaluated other molecular biomarkers such as neutrophil–lymphocyte ratio (NLR) and platelet/lymphocyte ratio (PLR), the higher the level, the worse the prognosis [40, 41], and the concentration of C-reactive protein (CRP) and cytokines such as TNF-alpha, IL-1 and others, whose increase is related to inflammatory aetiology [41–49].

Finally, as mentioned in chapter "MRI in Sudden Sensorineural Hearing", accumulating studies have confirmed that 3.0T MRI, especially the 3D-FLAIR sequence, has good sensitivity and specificity to the alterations in ISSNHL inner ear signals [15–20]. The application of 3D-FLAIR MRI can assist clinicians in finding different pathological changes in the inner ear on time. Therefore, 3D-FLAIR MRI has a potentially important clinical value for the possible pathological mechanism and prognosis assessment of ISSNHL. In a recent meta-analysis on 3D-FLAIR MRI to detect alterations in the inner ear of ISSNHL including eight studies and 638 patients, Lammers et al. [50] found that 29% of patients with ISSNHL had higher signal areas on 3D-FLAIR imaging, which suggests the pathological changes in the inner ear. Wang et al. [18] have found that there were significantly more patients with profound deafness in the inner ear haemorrhage group (72.47%) than in the normal group (23.82%), increased protein content group (53.47%) and BLB damage group (52.73%). Similarly, there were significantly more patients with total deafness in the inner ear haemorrhage group (71.56%) than in the normal group (16.37%), increased protein content group (53.13%) and BLB damage group (50.91%) (Fig. 4).

Thus, for our clinical practice, we can summarise that in ISSNHL there are five factors that affect prognosis: age, worse with older ages; type of audiometric curve, worse when high frequencies are affected; presence of vertigo, which worsens prognosis; delay in treatment, worse the later it starts; and, of course, severity, worse in hearing loss >50 dB. Also, MRI findings and biomarkers should be studied to determine the prognosis of each case (Table 2).

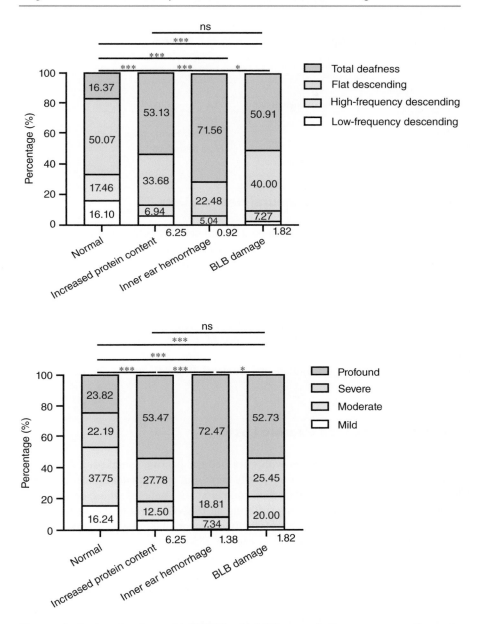

Fig. 4 Distribution of patients with ISSNHL with MRI pattern in four groups according to the degree of deafness (top) and type of deafness (bottom). *$p < 0.05$, ***$p < 0.001$, ns indicates no significance. (Reprinted with permission from: Wang M, Hu N, Wang Y, et al. Clinical value of 3D-FLAIR MRI in idiopathic sudden sensorineural hearing loss. ACS Chem Neurosci. 2022; 13: 151–7. Copyright (2022) American Chemical Society [18])

Table 2 Main prognostic factors in ISSNHL

	Impact on prognosis	
	Positive	Negative
Age	<60 years	>60 years
Delay to treatment	<7 days	>7 days
Pattern of hearing loss	Low frequency	Flat
Symptoms		Vertigo
MRI		Inner ear haemorrhage
Lab		High fibrinogen

Bilateral Sudden Sensorineural Hearing Loss

There have been descriptions of simultaneous bilateral ISSNHL of different aetiologies. Sara et al. [51] conducted a literature review, finding a total of 103 reported cases of bilateral SSNHL. The most frequent causes were toxic (29%), neoplastic (16%), vascular (16%) and autoimmune (16%), with it being essential to rule out systemic pathology in these cases [52–54].

However, bilateral cases are rare, accounting for only 0.5–5% of total ISSNHL. Xenellis et al. [55] reported the difference between cases of bilateral ISSNHL of simultaneous (with a difference of <3 days between one ear and the other) or sequential presentation. In their case series, out of a total of 232 cases of ISSNHL, there were 11 simultaneous bilateral ISSNHL and 7 sequential bilateral ISSNHL.

Sudden Single-Sided Hearing Loss

Fortunately, ISSNHL inpatients with only one ear hearing (single-sided deafness [SSD]) is a rare phenomenon. It obviously entails an even greater therapeutic challenge. Stahl and Cohen [56] found that, compared with patients whose contralateral hearing was normal, SSD patients suffering an ISSNHL went to the doctor earlier (2.8 vs 5.2 days) and responded similarly to treatment, obtaining an improvement of >10 dB in 50% of cases, and useful hearing in 60% of cases.

On the contrary, Liu et al. [57] also compared ISSNHL in SSD patients to normal contralateral ones. Initial hearing threshold showed no significant differences between the SSD group and the non-SSD group. Hearing gains and the rate of significant recovery were lower in the SSD group than in the non-SSD group.

However, both Cvoroviç et al. [22] and Hiraumi et al. [58] presented retrospective studies on 541 and 89 patients with ISSNHL, respectively, in which the condition of the contralateral ear is an important prognostic factor: when ISSNHL affected the best ear, the prognosis was worse. However, single-sided hearing loss that does not recover should receive a cochlear implant as soon as possible, ideally within 3–12 months of ISSNHL.

Current Recovery Criteria

One of the challenges within the assessment of SSNHL is to calculate the degree of recovery of these patients in audiometric terms, given that various criteria have been proposed by different authors, without any being universally accepted, which makes it very difficult to compare results [1–7, 59].

The best known in our field are Siegel's criteria [60]. This author proposed recovery criteria for SSNHL by dividing patients into four groups according to how many dB they improve (Table 3).

In the North American consensus of the AAO-HNS [4, 5], since 2012, the improvement of 10 dB in PTA of 0.5, 1 and 2 kHz has been accepted as one of the parameters for recovery, but Stachler's criteria are defined by incorporating the assessment of speech audiometry in all cases (Table 4). These criteria are maintained in the 2019 consensus review [5] and were adopted in the latest Spanish consensus review, also in 2019 [3].

In 2018, Cheng et al. [51] proposed a modification of Siegel's criteria, incorporating the concept of non-serviceable hearing, defined as average threshold loss >90 dB, as audioprosthetic adaptation is possible in other cases (Table 5).

Table 3 Siegel's ISSNHL recovery criteria (1975) [60]

Type		Hearing recovery
I	Complete recovery	Patients whose final hearing level is better than 25 dB, regardless of the size of the gain
II	Partial recovery	Patients who show >15 dB of gain and whose final hearing level is between 25 and 45 dB
III	Slight recovery	Patients who show >15 dB of gain and whose final hearing level is poorer than 45 dB
IV	No recovery	Patients who show <15 dB of gain and whose final hearing is poorer than 75 dB

Table 4 ISSNHL recovery criteria from Stachler et al. [4, 5]

Improvement	Pure tone audiometry	Speech audiometry
Complete recovery	Final PTA ≤ 10 dB HL of the previous threshold	SRT at most 5–10% worse than unaffected ear
Partial recovery	Improvement >10 dB of final PTA	Improvement >10% of SRT, without reaching complete recovery
No recovery	Improvement <10 dB of final PTA	Improvement <10% of SRT

SRT speech recognition score

Table 5 Modification of Siegel's ISSNHL recovery criteria taken from Cheng et al. [61]

Pre-treatment hearing levels	
Type 1	Mean threshold ≤25 dB
Type 2	Mean threshold 26–45 dB
Type 3	Mean threshold 46–75 dB
Type 4	Mean threshold 76–90 dB
Type 5	Mean threshold > 90 dB
Hearing recovery levels	
Complete recovery (CR)	Final hearing level ≤ 25 dB
Partial recovery (PR)	Patients who show >15 dB of gain and whose final hearing level is between 26 and 45 dB
Slight recovery (SR)	Patients who show >15 dB of gain and whose final hearing level is between 75 and 45 dB
No recovery (NR)	Patients who show >15 dB of gain and whose final hearing level is between 76 and 90 dB
Non-serviceable hearing (NSH)	Patients who show final hearing level > 90 dB

Long-Term Outcomes: Relapses

Most authors suggest monitoring SSNHL for at least 12 months to rule out relapses or progression to Ménière's disease. The possibility of a relapse is especially important when low frequencies are affected due to the possible progression to Ménière's disease, even if the SSNHL has presented without vertigo [6, 62].

In 2014, Wu et al. [63] conducted a study in Taiwan comparing two retrospective cohorts of 45,715 patients each, which were monitored for 3 years. One group of patients had had ISSNHL and the other had not. The cumulative incidence of ISSNHL relapse was up to 11.99 times higher than the incidence of an initial ISSNHL. Relapses were more frequent in patients over 60 years of age and with cardiovascular risk factors (hypertension, diabetes, etc.).

In 2018, Shi et al. [64] reviewed a series of 665 cases of ISSNHL, finding 12 relapses, in which the clearest risk factor was hyperlipidaemia, with a very high odds ratio (OR) (OR 54).

In a recent literature review including seven studies and 3781 patients, Zhang et al. [65] found 96 recurrent cases, with a recurrence rate of 1.4–7%, which mostly appear in the first two years after the initial SSNHL. The risk factors for recurrence are SSNHL affecting low frequencies, the association of tinnitus and the existence of high ratios of the neutrophil/lymphocyte and thrombocyte/lymphocyte ratio.

Early et al. [66] have done a case–control study comparing patients with ISSNHL to patients with non-sudden sensorineural hearing loss (SNHL). In patients with post-ISSNHL recovery to good hearing [PTA < 30 dB and word recognition score (WRS) > 70%], median time to progression to non-serviceable (PTA > 50 dB or WRS < 50%) SNHL was 16.4 years. Thus, patients should be counselled on continued risk to long-term hearing after stabilisation of hearing post-ISSNHL, with particular emphasis on greater risk to the contralateral ear in those with incomplete ipsilateral recovery.

Ko et al. [67] have shown that 6.7% (17,270/257,123) of the patients had at least one recurrence of SSNHL. The recurrence rate increases with the number of recurrences and over time. The recurrence rate appeared to decrease with age. Therefore, considerable efforts should be made to prevent recurrence.

Another Outcome Measure in ISSNHL: Improvement in Quality of Life

Having ISSNHL is a major loss of quality of life for patients that we need to be able to assess and remedy, as demonstrated in several studies [3, 5, 68–77].

Chiossoine-Kerdel et al. [68] reported the incidence of residual tinnitus after ISSNHL in 67% of cases, using the *Tinnitus Handicap Inventory* (THI) and *Hearing Handicap Inventory in Adults* (HHIA), with quality of life being significantly affected in 86% of patients.

It would be advisable to conduct both tests in each case of ISSNHL, at least, at the end of the treatment to see what repercussion the resulting hearing loss has, given that both are also validated in Spanish [69–71].

Carlsson et al. [73] studied a case series of 558 patients with ISSNHL through quality-of-life surveys. With a 63% response rate, sick leave was three times more frequent in these patients than in the general population, reflecting a lower quality of life when tinnitus or vertigo persisted after ISSNHL; yet they were not directly proportional to the degree of hearing loss.

Härkönen et al. [74] reviewed a case series of 217 patients with ISSNHL, 8 years after its onset. They studied their quality of life, hearing quality, stress level, presence of tinnitus and long-term impaired balance. They observed that quality of life and hearing was higher in cases where there was considered to be hearing recovery, and better still if there was no tinnitus or impaired balance. Over the years, the hearing impairment of the affected ear was similar to that of the healthy ear (6–7 dB).

Noguchi et al. [75] observed that, while improvement in pure tone audiometry is achieved before 3 months and remains stable, improvement in speech discrimination is later in 47% of cases, sometimes taking up to 12 months.

Sano et al. [76] published a multicentre study of 167 patients with ISSNHL assessing quality of life using the *Short Form Health Survey Version 2*. They observed how the mental component is affected at all ages, confirming that ISSNHL has a significant impact on patients' quality of life.

Sun et al. [77] conducted a clinical trial of 438 patients with ISSNHL, with one group being treated conventionally and the other receiving personalised psychological treatment. They observed that this individual treatment improved anxiety and depression surveys.

Conclusions

Due to the lack of evidence in the aetiology of SSNHL, there are still no conclusive prognostic factors to determine its progression. However, for our clinical practice, we can summarise that in ISSNHL there are five factors that affect prognosis: age, worse with older ages; type of audiometric curve, worse when high frequencies are affected; presence of vertigo, which worsens prognosis; delay in treatment, worse the later it starts; and, of course, severity, worse in hearing loss >50 dB.

The most used criteria in Spain for the assessment of recovery after an ISSNHL episode are Siegel's criteria, although the Spanish consensus of 2019 recommends using Stachler's criteria, which incorporate speech audiometry. However, the lack of consensus on the different recovery criteria used globally makes it difficult to compare studies.

The involvement of low frequencies or the presence of cardiovascular risk factors have been seen as risk factors for relapse.

The presence of associated symptoms, such as tinnitus or vertigo, can be predictors of poor quality of life, whereas recovery of social hearing is an excellent parameter of good quality of life.

References

1. Rauch SD. Clinical practice. Idiopathic sudden sensorineural hearing loss. N Engl J Med. 2008;359:833–40.
2. Plaza G, Durio E, Herráiz C, Asociación Madrileña de ORL, et al. Consenso sobre el diagnóstico y tratamiento de la sordera súbita. Acta Otorrinolaringol Esp. 2011;62:144–57.
3. Herrera M, García Berrocal JR, García Arumí A, et al. Update on consensus on diagnosis and treatment of idiopathic sudden sensorineural hearing loss. Acta Otorrinolaringol Esp (Engl Ed). 2019;70:290–300.
4. Stachler RJ, Chandrasekhar SS, Archer SM, American Academy of Otolaryngology-Head and Neck Surgery, et al. Clinical practice guideline: sudden hearing loss. Otolaryngol Head Neck Surg. 2012;146(Suppl. 3):S1–35.
5. Chandrasekhar SS, Tsai Do BS, Schwartz SR, et al. Clinical practice guideline: sudden hearing loss (update). Otolaryngol Head Neck Surg. 2019;161(Suppl. 1):S1–S45.
6. O'Connor Reina C, García Iriarte MT, Casado Morente JC, et al. Factores pronósticos en la sordera súbita. In: Plaza G, editor. Sordera súbita: diagnóstico y tratamiento. Madrid: Ergon; 2018. p. 151–60.
7. Mattox DE, Simmons FB. Natural history of sudden sensorineural hearing loss. Ann Otol Rhinol Laryngol. 1977;86:463–80.
8. Wilson WR, Byl FM, Laird N. The efficacy of steroids in the treatment of idiopathic sudden hearing loss. A double blind clinical study. Arch Otolaryngol. 1980;106:772–6.
9. Nosrati-Zarenoe R, Hultcrantz E. Corticosteroid treatment of idiopathic sudden sensorineural hearing loss: randomized triple-blind placebo-controlled trial. Otol Neurotol. 2012;33:523–31.
10. Bayoumy AB, van der Veen EL, Alexander de Ru J. Assessment of spontaneous recovery rates in patients with idiopathic sudden sensorineural hearing loss. JAMA Otolaryngol Head Neck Surg. 2018;144:655–6.
11. Chaushu H, Ungar OJ, Eta RA, et al. Spontaneous recovery rate of idiopathic sudden sensorineural hearing loss: a systematic review and meta-analysis. Clin Otolaryngol. 2023;48:395–402.

12. Wen YH, Chen PR, Wu HP. Prognostic factors of profound idiopathic sudden sensorineural hearing loss. Eur Arch Otorrinolaringol. 2014;271:1423–9.
13. Wei FQ, Wen L, Chen K, et al. Different prognoses in patients with profound sudden sensorineural hearing loss. Acta Otolaryngol. 2019;139:598–603.
14. Cho Y, Kim J, Oh SJ, et al. Clinical features and prognosis of severe-to-profound sudden sensorineural hearing loss. Am J Otolaryngol. 2022;43:103455.
15. Berrettini S, Seccia V, Fortunato S, et al. Analysis of the 3-dimensional fluid-attenuated inversion-recovery (3D-FLAIR) sequence in idiopathic sudden sensorineural hearing loss. JAMA Otolaryngol Head Neck Surg. 2013;139:456–64.
16. Chen K, Wen L, Zong L, et al. Audiological outcomes in sudden sensorineural hearing loss with presumed inner ear hemorrhage. Am J Otolaryngol. 2019;40:274–8.
17. Arellano B, Brea B, Gonzalez FM. Labyrinthine haemorrhage secondary to oral anticoagulants. Acta Otorrinolaringol Esp. 2016;67:185–6.
18. Wang M, Hu N, Wang Y, et al. Clinical value of 3D-FLAIR MRI in idiopathic sudden sensorineural hearing loss. ACS Chem Neurosci. 2022;13:151–7.
19. Compagnone L, Levigne V, Pereira B, et al. Injected 3T-3D-FLAIR-MRI labyrinthine patterns match with the severity and tonotopic alteration in sudden sensorineural hearing loss. Eur Arch Otorrinolaringol. 2022;279:4883–91.
20. Conte G, Di Berardino F, Mastrapasqua RF, et al. Prognostic value of early magnetic resonance imaging patterns in sudden hearing loss. Audiol Neurootol. 2022;27:64–74.
21. Mattox DE, Lyles CA. Idiopathic sudden sensorineural hearing loss. Am J Otol. 1989;10:242–7.
22. Cvorović L, Deric D, Probst R, Hegemann S. Prognostic model for predicting hearing recovery in idiopathic sudden sensorineural hearing loss. Otol Neurotol. 2008;29:464–9.
23. Bing D, Ying J, Miao J, et al. Predicting the hearing outcome in sudden sensorineural hearing loss via machine learning models. Clin Otolaryngol. 2018;43:868–74.
24. Shimanuki MN, Shinden S, Oishi N, et al. Early hearing improvement predicts the prognosis of idiopathic sudden sensorineural hearing loss. Eur Arch Otorrinolaringol. 2021;278:4251–8.
25. Lin W, Xiong G, Yan K, et al. Clinical features and influencing factors for the prognosis of patients with sudden deafness. Front Neurol. 2022;13:905069.
26. Lee MK, Jeon ET, Baek N, et al. Prediction of hearing recovery in unilateral sudden sensorineural hearing loss using artificial intelligence. Sci Rep. 2022;12:3977.
27. Zhou W, Yuan H, et al. Nomogram for predicting the prognostic role in idiopathic sudden sensorineural hearing loss. Am J Otolaryngol. 2023;44:103736.
28. Wu H, Wan W, Jiang H, Xiong Y. Prognosis of idiopathic sudden sensorineural hearing loss: the nomogram perspective. Ann Otol Rhinol Laryngol. 2023;132:5–12.
29. Aghakhani A, Yousefi M, Yekaninejad MS. Machine learning models for predicting sudden sensorineural hearing loss outcome: a systematic review. Ann Otol Rhinol Laryngol. 2024;133(3):268–76.
30. Uhm TW, Yi S, et al. Hearing recovery prediction and prognostic factors of idiopathic sudden sensorineural hearing loss: a retrospective analysis with a deep neural network model. Braz J Otorhinolaryngol. 2023;89:101273.
31. Huang GJ, Luo MS, Lu BQ, Li SH. Noninvasive prognostic factors and web predictive tools for idiopathic sudden sensorineural hearing loss. Am J Otolaryngol. 2023;44:103965.
32. Panda NK, Verma RK, Saravanan K. Sudden sensorineural hearing loss: have we got a cure? J Otolaryngol Head Neck Surg. 2008;37:807–12.
33. Jung WW, Hoegerl C. Sudden sensorineural hearing loss and why it's an emergency. Cureus. 2022;14:e21418.
34. Chen I, Eligal S, Menahem O, et al. Time from sudden sensory neural hearing loss to treatment as a prognostic factor. Front Neurol. 2023;14:1158955.
35. Klein L, Handzel O, Shilo S, et al. Is sudden sensorineural hearing loss an otologic emergency? Evidence-Based cutoff for optimal treatment initiation for sudden unilateral sensorineural hearing loss: a case series and meta-analyses. Otol Neurotol. 2023;44:216–22.

36. Amarillo E, Navarro A, Hernández-García E, Plaza G. Intratympanic steroids for combined treatment of idiopathic sudden hearing loss: when is it too late? Acta Otolaryngol. 2019;139:632–5.
37. Kanzaki S, Sakagami M, Hosoi H, et al. High fibrinogen in peripheral blood correlates with poorer hearing recovery in idiopathic sudden sensorineural hearing loss. PLoS One. 2014;9:e104680.
38. Okuda H, Aoki M, Ohashi T, et al. Serum fibrinogen level and cytokine production as prognostic biomarkers for idiopathic sudden sensorineural hearing loss. Otol Neurotol. 2022;43:e712–9.
39. Oya R, Takenaka Y, Imai T, et al. Serum fibrinogen as a prognostic factor in sudden sensorineural hearing loss: a meta-analysis. Otol Neurotol. 2018;39:e929–5.
40. Kang JW, Kim MG, Kim SS, et al. Neutrophil-lymphocyte ratio as a valuable prognostic marker in idiopathic sudden sensorineural hearing loss. Acta Otolaryngol. 2020;140:307–13.
41. Ni W, Song SP, Jiang YD. Association between routine hematological parameters and sudden sensorineural hearing loss: a meta-analysis. J Otol. 2021;16:47–54.
42. Diao T, Ke Y, Zhang J, Jing Y, Ma X. Correlation between the prognosis of sudden total deafness and the peripheral blood inflammation markers. Front Neurol. 2022;13:927235.
43. Sun H, Jiang W, Wang J. The prognostic value of peripheral blood parameters on all-frequency sudden sensorineural hearing loss. Braz J Otorhinolaryngol. 2023;89:101302.
44. Zhang X, Wang Y, Yan Q, et al. Prognostic Correlation of immune-inflammatory markers in sudden sensorineural hearing loss: a retrospective study. Ear Nose Throat J. 2023:1455613231202498.
45. Al-Azzawi A, Stapleton E. Blood tests as biomarkers for the diagnosis and prognosis of sudden sensorineural hearing loss in adults: a systematic review. J Laryngol Otol. 2023;137:977–84.
46. Song J, Ouyang F, Xiong Y, et al. Reassessment of oxidative stress in idiopathic sudden hearing loss and preliminary exploration of the effect of physiological concentration of melatonin on prognosis. Front Neurol. 2023;14:1249312.
47. Zhou T, Chen M, Yuan Z, et al. Inflammatory markers and the risk of idiopathic sudden sensorineural hearing loss: a Mendelian randomization study. Front Neurol. 2023;14:1111255.
48. Niknazar S, Bazgir N, Shafaei V, et al. Assessment of prognostic biomarkers in sudden sensorineural hearing loss: a systematic review and meta-analysis. Clin Biochem. 2023;121–122:110684.
49. Cavallaro G, Pantaleo A, Pontillo V, et al. endothelial dysfunction and metabolic disorders in patients with sudden sensorineural hearing loss. Medicina (Kaunas). 2023;59:1718.
50. Lammers MJW, Young E, Fenton D, et al. The prognostic value and pathophysiologic significance of three-dimensional fluid-attenuated inversion recovery (3D-FLAIR) magnetic resonance imaging in idiopathic sudden sensorineural hearing loss: a systematic review and meta-analysis. Clin Otolaryngol. 2019;44:1017–25.
51. Sara SA, Teh BM, Friedland P. Bilateral sudden sensorineural hearing loss: review. J Laryngol Otol. 2014;128(Suppl. 1):S8–15.
52. Metrailer AM, Babu SC. Management of sudden sensorineural hearing loss. Curr Opin Otolaryngol Head Neck Surg. 2016;24:403–6.
53. Elias TGA, Monsanto RDC, Jean LS, et al. Bilateral sudden sensorineural hearing loss: a distinct phenotype entity. Otol Neurotol. 2022;43:437–42.
54. Wang Y, Xiong W, Sun X, et al. Characteristics and prognosis analysis of bilateral sudden sensorineural hearing loss: a retrospective case-control study. Clin Otolaryngol. 2022;47:732–40.
55. Xenellis J, Nikolopoulos TP, Stavroulaki P, et al. Simultaneous and sequential bilateral sudden sensorineural hearing loss: are they different from unilateral sudden sensorineural hearing loss? ORL J Otorhinolaryngol Relat Spec. 2007;69:306–10.
56. Stahl N, Cohen D. Idiopathic sudden sensorineural hearing loss in the only hearing ear: patient characteristics and hearing outcome. Arch Otolaryngol Head Neck Surg. 2006;132:193–5.
57. Liu Y, Wu W, Li S, et al. Clinical characteristics and prognosis of sudden sensorineural hearing loss in single-sided deafness patients. Front Neurol. 2023;14:1230340.

58. Hiraumi H, Yamamoto N, Sakamoto T, Ito J. Multivariate analysis of hearing outcomes in patients with idiopathic sudden sensorineural hearing loss. Acta Otolaryngol Suppl. 2010;563:24–8.
59. O'Malley MR, Haynes DS. Sudden hearing loss. Otolaryngol Clin N Am. 2008;41:633–49.
60. Siegel LG. The treatment of idiopathic sudden sensorineural hearing loss. Otolaryngol Clin N Am. 1975;8:467–73.
61. Cheng YF, Chu YC, Tu TY, et al. Modified Siegel's criteria for sudden sensorineural hearing loss: reporting recovery outcomes with matched pretreatment hearing grades. J Chin Med Assoc. 2018;81:1008–12.
62. Yoshida T, Sone M, Kitoh R, et al. Idiopathic sudden sensorineural hearing loss and acute low-tone sensorineural hearing loss: a comparison of the results of a nationwide epidemiological survey in Japan. Acta Otolaryngol. 2017;137(Suppl. 565):S38–43.
63. Wu CM, Lee KJ, Chang SL, et al. Recurrence of idiopathic sudden sensorineural hearing loss: a retrospective cohort study. Otol Neurotol. 2014;35:1736–41.
64. Shi WY, Li KJ, Li Q. Analysis of risk factors for recurrent sudden sensorineural hearing loss. Lin Chung Er Bi Yan Hou Tou Jing Wai Ke Za Zhi. 2018;32:976–8.
65. Zhang BY, Wang YC, Chan KC. Recurrent sudden sensorineural hearing loss—a literature review. Laryngosc Investig Otolaryngol. 2022;7:854–62.
66. Early S, van der Valk JC, Frijns JHM, Stankovic KM. Accelerated long-term hearing loss progression after recovery from idiopathic sudden sensorineural hearing loss. Front Neurol. 2021;12:738942.
67. Ko HY, Nam HJ, Kim MH. A nationwide population-based study for the recurrence and comorbidities in sudden sensorineural hearing loss. Laryngoscope. 2024;134(3):1417–25.
68. Chiossoine-Kerdel JA, Baguley DM, Stoddart RL, Moffat DA. An investigation of the audiologic handicap associated with unilateral sudden sensorineural hearing loss. Am J Otol. 2000;21:645–51.
69. Newman CW, Jacobson GP, Spitzer JB. Development of the tinnitus handicap inventory. Arch Otolaryngol Head Neck Surg. 1996;122:143–8.
70. Newman CW, Weinstein BE, Jacobson GP, Hug GA. the hearing handicap inventory for adults: psychometric adequacy and audiometric correlates. Ear Hear. 1990;11:430–3.
71. Herraiz C, Hernández Calvín J, Plaza G, et al. Evaluación de la incapacidad en pacientes con acúfenos. Acta Otorrinolaringol Esp. 2001;52:534–8.
72. Carrillo A, Medina MDM, Polo R, et al. Validation of the hearing handicap inventory for adults scale for Spanish-speaking patients. Otol Neurotol. 2019;40:e947–54.
73. Carlsson PI, Hall M, Lind KJ, Danermark B. Quality of life, psychosocial consequences, and audiological rehabilitation after sudden sensorineural hearing loss. Int J Audiol. 2011;50:139–44.
74. Härkönen K, Kivekäs I, Rautiainen M, et al. Quality of life and hearing eight years after sudden sensorineural hearing loss. Laryngoscope. 2017;127:927–31.
75. Noguchi Y, Takahashi M, Ito T, et al. Delayed restoration of maximum speech discrimination scores in patients with idiopathic sudden sensorineural hearing loss. Auris Nasus Larynx. 2016;43:495–500.
76. Sano H, Okamoto M, Ohhashi K, et al. Quality of life reported by patients with idiopathic sudden sensorineural hearing loss. Otol Neurotol. 2013;34:36–40.
77. Sun B, Liu L, Ren X, Wang Z. Psychological state of patients with sudden deafness and the effect of psychological intervention on recovery. J Int Med Res. 2020;48:300060520957536.

Treatment of Idiopathic Sudden Sensorineural Hearing Loss with Systemic Corticosteroids

Guillermo Plaza, Antonio Lara Peinado, Marta Alcaraz Fuentes, and José Ramón García Berrocal

Introduction

After the introduction in the 1970s of the use of corticosteroids in autoimmune diseases [1, 2], the first papers that applied them in idiopathic sudden sensorineural hearing loss (ISSNHL) were presented in the 1980s [3–6]. Of these, it was the famous clinical trial published by Wilson et al. [5] in 1980 that led to their widespread use in ISSNHL [7, 8], accepted as the gold standard treatment ever since [9–12].

In fact, in a condition such as ISSNHL, characterised by an unknown aetiology, an uncertain pathophysiology and a high spontaneous recovery rate, empirical treatment with systemic corticosteroids, even at high doses, is tempting to apply, but also highly criticised by many authors [8, 13–15].

However, although nearly all otolaryngologists currently treat ISSNHL with corticosteroids, there is much variability in their use in ISSNHL. Thus, various surveys among ENT specialists describe the lack of uniformity in the use of systemic corticosteroids in ISSNHL: in the route of administration, oral or intravenous; in the

G. Plaza (✉)
Ear, Nose and Throat Department, Hospital Universitario de Fuenlabrada, Madrid, Spain

Ear, Nose and Throat Department, Hospital Universitario Sanitas La Zarzuela, Madrid, Spain

Universidad Rey Juan Carlos, Madrid, Spain
e-mail: guillermo.plaza@salud.madrid.org

A. Lara Peinado · M. Alcaraz Fuentes
Ear, Nose and Throat Department, Hospital Universitario Sanitas La Zarzuela, Madrid, Spain

J. R. García Berrocal
Ear, Nose and Throat Department, Hospital Universitario Puerto de Hierro, Majadahonda, Madrid, Spain

Universidad Autónoma de Madrid, Madrid, Spain

G. Plaza, J. R. García Berrocal (eds.), *Sudden Sensorineural Hearing Loss*, https://doi.org/10.1007/978-3-031-61385-2_7

dose, prednisone from 20 to 60 mg/day; in duration, from 5 to 30 days; or in the chosen drug, whether prednisone, deflazacort or others [16]. This diversity of protocols makes comparisons of results very difficult, and a critical analysis of them is necessary.

Oral Corticosteroids in ISSNHL

After the publication of the abovementioned randomised clinical trial by Wilson et al. [5] in 1980, only case series were reported for 25 years, generally reinforcing the empirical use of oral corticosteroids in ISSNHL, without reviewing this work in detail.

The three most relevant studies in these years are retrospective. On the one hand, in Japan, Minoda et al. [17] presented in 2000 a retrospective series of 255 patients with ISSNHL treated with oral prednisone, observing that, paradoxically, those who received >30 mg/day of prednisone had worse auditory response. These authors went as far as to not recommend the initial treatment of all ISSNHL with steroids. On the other hand, in the retrospective review carried out by Chen et al. [18] in 2003 at Harvard University, tonal and verbal audiometry results were analysed in a sample of 318 patients treated for over 10 years. In comparing patients treated with oral corticosteroids and patients who refused treatment, a significant improvement was found in the treated group, which also initially had severe hearing loss. Finally, Slattery et al. [19], at the House Ear Institute in California, published in 2005 another retrospective review of 75 patients who were treated within the first 2 weeks of symptom onset with doses up to 60 mg of prednisone daily. On analysing the results in tonal and verbal audiometry exams, patients treated with high doses (60 mg/day) responded better than patients treated with lower doses or who were treated later.

The arrival of the school of thought of evidence-based medicine initially saw systematic reviews and meta-analyses being published that comprehensively reviewed the published works [20–22], including the only two randomised clinical trials: those published by Wilson et al. [5] and Cinamon et al. [23], which were thoroughly reviewed and critiqued [15, 22]. According to these meta-analyses, oral corticosteroids should no longer be considered the gold standard treatment due to the severe limitations of the studies that support their use (low number of patients per group, variability in definition of ISSNHL, different treatment plans, different outcomes that were measured at different times after treatment). In fact, a favourable odds ratio (OR) was obtained for the use oral corticosteroids, but it was not significant (OR 2.47; 95% CI 0.89–6.84) (Table 1).

These reviews thoroughly analysed the classic work by Wilson et al. [5], which is the most cited by all experts. It was a double-blind, randomised clinical trial. To measure results, authors at that time would use the healthy ear, using as a reference the so-called recovery rate, which was considered full with a difference within 10 dB, partial with a recovery greater than 50% with respect to the healthy ear or none if there was less than 50% recovery. With these premises, a hearing recovery

Table 1 Pooled data from the three randomised oral corticosteroid clinical trials compared to placebo showed no differences between treatment groups in both meta-analyses from Conlin and Parnes [22] and Crane et al. [28]

	Steroids	Placebo	OR (95%)	Significance
Wilson et al. [5]	20/33	11/34	3.22 (1.18–8.76)	Yes
Cinamon et al. [23]	8/10	9/11	0.89 (0.10–7.86)	No
Total from Conlin and Parnes [21]			**2.47 (0.89–6.84)**	**No**
Nosrati-Zarenoe [25]	18/47	18/46	0.97 (0.42–2.22)	No
Total from Crane et al. [28]			**1.52 (0.83–2.77)**	**No**

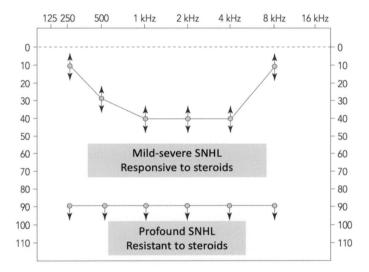

Fig. 1 Categories of ISSNHL, modified from Wilson et al. [5]: from profound hearing loss, unresponsive to oral corticosteroids, to mild medium-frequency hearing loss with good response

rate was obtained in 61% of the group that received steroid treatment compared to 32% of the patients in the placebo group; that is, treating ISSNHL with corticosteroids implied a probability of improvement up to 4.3 times greater. In addition, all patients with medium-frequency loss fully recovered hearing, while 76% of patients with profound loss did not recover hearing, stratifying ISSNHL by severity. There were no significant adverse effects associated with oral corticosteroids (Fig. 1).

Recently, Song et al. [24] critically reviewed Wilson's paper, concluding that it was not truly randomised, had important selection bias, did not perform a proper power analysis, included different drugs and dosages in distinct hospitals, and selectively withheld study drug from certain participants based on early study results, amplifying selection bias. The study's conclusion that steroids have a 'definite positive effect' on hearing recovery was overstated given the multiple issues with the study design (Fig. 2).

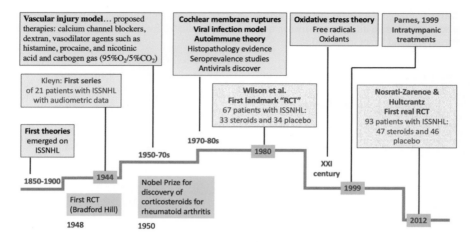

Fig. 2 The rise and fall of steroids in ISSNHL. After starting to be used in 1970, the landmark paper by Wilson et al. in 1980 resulted in steroids as the mainstay treatment in ISSNHL, until 2012 when Nosrati-Zarenoe's RTC showed a lack of significant effect, at the same time as intratympanic therapy started

It took 30 years until Nosrati-Zarenoe and Hultcrantz [25] published a randomised, triple-blind clinical trial in 2012, including 93 patients treated with prednisolone, at doses of 1 mg/kg/day, or placebo. They concluded that oral corticosteroids at usual doses do not seem to influence the hearing recovery of patients with ISSNHL, as recovery was full in 40% of patients in both groups, partial in 46% with corticosteroids and 38% without them, which were non-significant differences. Subsequently, in 2015, the same authors [26] presented a comparative analysis of their trial with data from the Swedish database on ISSNHL, in which there was a group of patients who did not receive any treatment, neither pharmacological nor placebo. After this analysis, again, oral corticosteroids were not superior to placebo as the improvement in dB was very similar (36 ± 22 dB vs. 30 ± 24 dB, respectively). These discouraging results broke the myth of the effectiveness of oral corticosteroids in ISSNHL.

This has led to the publication of new systematic reviews and meta-analyses [27, 28], among which the one presented by Crane et al. [28] in 2015 stands out. After reviewing the three published trials, these authors concluded that there were no significant differences between the use of systemic corticosteroids and placebo, as an overall OR of 1.52 (95% CI 0.83–2.77) was obtained (Table 1).

More recently, Maldonado et al. [29] conducted a new review of the three ISSNHL trials that include placebo (Table 2). These authors suggested that a new study comparing oral corticosteroids with placebo is needed in order to better determine their actual effectiveness.

Due to these highly critical analyses, for many authors oral corticosteroids are no longer a mandatory treatment for ISSNHL. In fact, the North American consensus in 2019 [12] considered that they 'can be used' as a primary treatment, not that they

Table 2 Comparison of clinical trials comparing oral steroids and placebo in ISSNHL, modified from Maldonado et al. [29]

	Wilson et al. [5]	Cinamon et al. [23]	Nosrati-Zarenoe and Hultcrantz [25]
Sample size	33/34/56.0.123	21/41	93/103
Groups	Placebo Non-treatment	Placebo	Placebo
Limitations	Poor randomisation, merging placebo and non-treatment, and combining two hospitals with different drugs	Alternate randomisation, inadequate	Good randomisation, double-blind, does not meet intention to treat

'should be used' in all cases. Being optional, some ENT may not start treatment with steroids for some cases of ISSNHL.

Meanwhile, the Spanish consensus [10] recommended treating all cases of ISSNHL if they are diagnosed in the first 45 days after the onset of the episode. Three alternatives of corticosteroid treatment should be evaluated, with it being up to the specialist and depending on the concomitant disease of the patient to choose which one: the oral route, single primary intratympanic treatment or combined treatment (see chapter "Treatment of Idiopathic Sudden Sensorineural Hearing Loss with Intratympanic Corticosteroids").

Guidelines for the Administration of Oral Corticosteroids in ISSNHL

Classical pharmacological studies establish that the optimal doses to obtain the maximum benefit in acute inflammations should be prednisone at 1 mg/kg/day, administered in a single daily dose, and with a treatment period of at least 10–14 days, with the descending pattern being recommended to reduce the risk of secondary adrenal insufficiency [8–12, 30].

For ISSNHL, there is no single guideline, but an adequate guideline for oral corticosteroids would be to administer maximum doses for 4 days, followed by a decrease of 10 mg every 2 days [7, 18]. To choose the correct dose, the equivalent dose of prednisolone with the other corticosteroids used should be taken into account: 60 mg of prednisone is equivalent to 48 mg of methylprednisolone and 10 mg of dexamethasone. If these proportions are not taken into account, it is easy to underdose. Starting treatment as early as possible is just as important as using the right dosage [8, 29]. The usual guideline is to administer them in the morning to respect the circadian rhythm [29–31].

According to Spanish consensus in 2019 [10], the recommended oral corticosteroid regimen in ISSNHL would be to administer a daily dose in the morning of 1 mg/kg of prednisone for 5 days, followed by a descending series for a total of 25 days.

High-Dose Systemic Corticosteroids (Pulses) in ISSNHL

Although the usual guideline recommended in consensus [10, 12] refers to oral corticosteroids, some authors suggest the use of corticosteroids at very high doses administered intermittently and intravenously, also known as pulses or megadoses. Widely used in inflammatory and rheumatic pathology, pulse treatment is defined as discontinuous intravenous administration of high doses of corticosteroids, with doses of more than 250 mg of prednisone per day, or its equivalents, for one or more days [32, 33].

In 2001, Alexiou et al. [34] published a case series of 603 patients with ISSNHL, of which one group was treated with rheological agents and another with rheological agents and prednisolone at daily doses of 500–1000 mg. These authors found a higher rate of hearing improvement in the group treated with corticosteroid pulses, while also significant for low and medium frequencies, so they recommend their use.

Niedermeyer et al. [35] showed that the level of cortisol in human perilymph was significantly higher after 250 mg intravenous prednisolone compared to 125 mg dose. The latter group had cortisol levels similar to the controls, who did not receive steroids. This was the initial rationale to introduce high-dose systemic steroids in German guidelines. Subsequently, other authors published the use of corticosteroid pulses as treatment of ISSNHL for at least three consecutive days [36–44] (Table 3). None of these studies can conclude that high doses of corticosteroids improve the prognosis for hearing recovery. Only the study by Narozny et al. [36] reported better auditory results in the group treated with pulses of 1 g of methylprednisolone per day for 3 days and hyperbaric oxygen, but the group not receiving pulses also did not receive hyperbaric oxygen, making it difficult to analyse the results. There is also some evidence from retrospective and prospective studies regarding treatment advantage for high-dose systemic steroids therapy [37–41].

However, Westerlaken et al. [42] conducted a randomised clinical trial on ISSNHL in which they compared a group treated with daily intravenous dexamethasone pulses of 300 mg for 3 days, followed by 4 days of placebo, with another group treated with 70 mg of oral prednisone in descending series for 7 days, without finding differences in hearing improvement between the two groups. The randomised clinical trial conducted by Eftekharian et al. [43], with 67 patients diagnosed with ISSNHL, compared one group treated with daily pulses of 500 mg methylprednisolone for 3 days, followed by oral prednisolone (1 mg/kg/day) for 11 days, with another group treated with oral prednisolone (1 mg/kg/day) for 14 days, but no

Table 3 Doses used as intravenous corticosteroid pulses in ISSNHL for at least three consecutive days

Alexiou et al. [34]	500–1000 mg prednisolone
Narozny et al. [36]	1 g methylprednisolone
Aoki et al. [37]	1200 mg hydrocortisone
Westerlaken et al. [42]	300 mg dexamethasone
Eftekharian et al. [43]	500 mg methylprednisolone
AMORL Consensus [9]	500 mg methylprednisolone

significant differences were found in terms of hearing recovery between the two groups.

Balai et al. [44] systematically reviewed all these six studies, representing 919 patients. Two prospective single-arm studies of patients with ISSNHL treated with a high-dose steroid regime found mean hearing level improved (79.5 dB to 42.3 dB) and 45.8% of idiopathic patients had complete recovery of hearing. Three retrospective case series comparing high-dose to standard-dose regimes found a significantly greater improvement in hearing level (38.3 dB vs. 48.8 dB), a greater mean absolute hearing gain (44.4 dB vs. 15.1 dB) and a significantly higher rate of functionally relevant recovery (35.7% vs. 7.4%) in patients treated with high-dose regimes. As mentioned, the single included prospective randomised trial.(4 [2]) found no statistically significant difference in the mean hearing level or speech discrimination score between patients treated with high-dose pulse steroids or a standard-dose regimen.

In some countries such as Japan or Germany, the usual pattern of systemic corticosteroids in ISSNHL is intravenous and high dose, at 200–250 mg/day [33, 45]. For instance, in the clinical guideline for ISSNHL in Germany, intravenous treatment with prednisolone at initial doses of 250 mg/day (range 100–500 mg/day), followed by a descending series, has been recommended since 2001 [46, 47]. A large clinical trial in Germany has just been concluded. The authors found that systemic high-dose glucocorticoid therapy was not superior to a lowerdose regimen in patients with ISSNHL, and it was associated with a higher risk of side effects [48].

Kovacs et al. [49] reported recently an RCT including 78 patients comparing the efficacy of high-dose systemic versus combined (systemic and intratympanic) corticosteroid therapy in ISSNHL. No differences were detected regarding hearing improvement between the two groups, based on any criteria. Coexisting cardiovascular comorbidity, vertigo and severity of the initial hearing loss may bear a significantly higher impact upon hearing improvement than the additional intratympanic steroid administration.

In Spain, the Association of Otolaryngology of Madrid (AMORL) published its consensus on the diagnosis and treatment of ISSNHL [9] in late 2010 and proposed the treatment with pulses of 500 mg of methylprednisolone per day for 7 days for severe single-side ISSNHL (> 70 dB) or ISSNHL with associated intense vertigo. This recommendation was maintained in the 2019 to present version of the Spanish consensus review [10].

Oral Corticosteroids as Adjunctive Therapy in ISSNHL

Although steroids are the mainstay for treatment of ISSNHL following current guidelines, in some countries other therapies are commonly used as adjunctive to them.

Ginkgo Biloba Extract

In Korea or China, Ginkgo biloba extract (GBE) is frequently used together with steroids as adjunctive treatment of ISSNHL [50, 51]. GBE is a traditional Chinese medicine preparation extracted from Ginkgo biloba dried leaves, with the effects of promoting blood circulation and removing blood stasis, activating the collaterals. It has the effect of improving inner ear circulation, preventing platelet aggregation and thrombosis, reducing blood viscosity and improving blood rheology, and exerting significant antioxidant activity, which can improve the activity of superoxide dismutase, accelerate the scavenging of oxygen-free radicals caused by ischaemia and protect cell tissues.

Koo et al. [50] presented an RCT comparing patients receiving a systemic steroid adding GBE or placebo. There was no difference in hearing improvement in PTA, but speech discrimination scores were better in the GBE group (69.17 ± 40.89 and $87.48 \pm 28.65\%$). Yuan et al. [51] published a meta-analysis including 27 articles with a total of 2623 patients with ISSNHL treated with GBE. The results revealed that the effects of GBE adjuvant therapy were superior to oral steroids (total effective rate: $RR = 1.22$, 95% CI: 1.18–1.26).

N-Acetylcysteine

In some geographical areas, it is common to add *N*-acetylcysteine (NAC) to oral steroids as the treatment of ISSNHL [52–57]. NAC has several effects that are thought to be beneficial to cell stress in the inner ear. Oxygenated radicals can damage hair cells in the inner ear by activating apoptotic cell death programs. NAC acts as a free radical scavenger and can decrease the cell's nitric oxide production by increasing the synthesis of reduced glutathione, thus decreasing the production of harmful nitrogen radicals.

Angeli et al. [52], from Miami (the United States), reported a case–control study of adult patients with ISSNHL, treated with oral prednisone plus intratympanic dexamethasone either alone or in combination with NAC. Higher gains at 4 kHz were noted with NAC use. The percentage of patients with at least 50% recovery was 63% and 35% for the combination and single-therapy groups, respectively. Chen et al. [53], from Taiwan, also presented a case–control study including patients with ISSNHL treated only with NAC versus those treated with corticosteroids and plasma expander. The NAC group showed significantly greater mean hearing gain than the other group (43 ± 27 dB vs. 21 ± 28 dB) and revealed better improved rate of hearing than group B (91% vs. 57%).

From Taiwan, Chen et al. [54] described a retrospective study on ISSNHL where the only significant difference between the NAC and non-NAC groups was the post-treatment pure tone audiometry (PTA) thresholds at 8 kHz, which were 54.2 ± 24.4 and 60.9 ± 34.1 dB, respectively. In China, Bai et al. [55] reported an RCT on ISSNHL showing that NAC combined with dexamethasone can effectively protect hair cells from oxidative stress. Again, a significant hearing gain at 8 kHz was observed in the NAC group. Moreover, the hearing recovery rates of the NAC group were much higher than that in the control group. Later, Bai et al. [56] published a meta-analysis including seven articles with a total of 1197 patients with SNHL (sudden or not) treated with NAC. Only two studies reported data for ISSNHL, showing that NAC improved patient outcomes of hearing tests in cases of ISSNHL, but did not prevent hearing loss induced by noise or ototoxicity.

More recently, in Germany, Kouka et al. [57] published a retrospective study on 793 patients with ISSNHL. A total of 663 patients were treated with NAC in addition to standard tapered prednisolone treatment. In multivariable analysis, significant negative prognosis of hearing recovery was age > median (odds ratio [OR] 1.648; 95% confidence interval [CI] 1.139–2.385), diseased opposite ear (OR 3.049; CI 2.157–4.310), pantonal ISSHL (OR 1.891; CI 1.309–2.732) and prednisolone alone without NAC treatment (OR 1.862; CI 1.200–2.887). Thus, prednisolone treatment combined with NAC resulted in better hearing outcomes in patients with ISSHL than treatment without NAC. For a better understanding of the role of NAC in the treatment of ISSNHL, clinical studies for the prospective design are needed to provide adequate evidence.

Side Effects of Systemic Corticosteroids in ISSNHL

As for the side effects of corticosteroids, the most dangerous is the suppression of the hypothalamic–pituitary–adrenal axis. However, it is uncommon for this to occur in the treatment of ISSNHL, given the usual dose and oral administration, if administered at the appropriate dose and time [32].

In the meta-analysis by Hoes et al. [58], although they vary according to the underlying condition, the most frequent side effects of corticosteroids (Table 4) are insomnia, mood disorders and behavioural disorders (20%), gastrointestinal disorders (15%), dermatological disorders (12%), neurological disorders (10%), weight gain and hyperglycaemia. The most severe, though rare, side effects are pancreatitis, bleeding, high blood pressure, cataracts, myopathy, opportunistic infections, osteoporosis and osteonecrosis [59–61].

Of these effects, the most common is hyperglycaemia, which can be complicated in patients with previous diabetes. Rohrmeier et al. [62] analysed hyperglycaemia secondary to systemic treatment with high-dose corticosteroids in ISSNHL and other conditions, observing that it was more frequent when the cumulative dose of prednisolone was >1500 mg, reaching detection in 67% of non-diabetic patients and 100% of diabetics. In other words, when megadoses or steroid pulses are used, the risk of side effects rises exponentially.

Halevy et al. [63] described that about one-third of ISSNHL patients treated with systemic corticosteroids discontinue treatment due to adverse effects, primarily hyperglycaemia and high blood pressure. Furthermore, this is more likely if there is prior diabetes or high blood pressure.

Table 4 Side effects of systemic corticosteroids

Musculoskeletal	Osteoporosis
	Osteonecrosis
	Myopathy
Metabolic–endocrinal	Glucose intolerance
	Diabetes
	Redistribution of fat and weight gain
	Sex hormone disorders
Cardiovascular	Dyslipidaemia
	Atherosclerosis
	Cardiovascular disease
	Oedema
	Heart failure
	Renal impairment
	High blood pressure
Dermatological	Skin atrophy
	Acne
	Hirsutism
	Alopecia
Ophthalmological	Cataracts
	Glaucoma
Gastrointestinal	Peptic ulcer
	Pancreatitis
Infection	Viral or bacterial infections
	Immunosuppression
Psychological	Mood disorders
	Steroid psychosis
Neurological	Headache
	Vertigo and instability
	Tinnitus

Attempts have been made to reduce the side effects of oral steroids by multiple divided daily doses instead of a single dose [64–66]. However, Yu et al. [65] showed that hearing improved significantly after a single-dose regimen.

Administration of corticosteroids should be avoided in patients with insulin-dependent diabetes mellitus, poorly controlled diabetics, labile hypertension, tuberculosis, peptic ulcer or prior psychotic reactions to corticosteroids. Another side effect that should be avoided is corticosteroid-induced osteoporosis, following the guidelines of the Spanish Society of Internal Medicine, adding calcium and/or vitamin D supplements when the use is prolonged [8, 32].

Conclusions

Although there are no solid studies linking the benefits of systemic corticosteroids against their side effects in ISSNHL, there is also insufficient evidence to conclude that treatment is ineffective. In fact, Cochrane reviews found no data favourable to the use of systemic corticosteroids in ISSNHL [20, 27], nor for antivirals and vasodilators.

Considering the huge impact of ISSNHL on the quality of life and the equally huge impact of an improvement in hearing, even if it is not complete, the administration of systemic corticosteroids is a reasonable treatment to offer to patients [7–12, 67], hence it is the usual treatment of this condition today. The correct design of new randomised studies may confirm this indication.

According to the current Spanish consensus on ISSNHL from 2019 [10], the recommended oral corticosteroid regimen in ISSNHL would be to administer a daily dose in the morning of 1 mg/kg of prednisone for 5 days, followed by a descending series for a total of 25 days.

References

1. McCabe BF. Autoimmune sensorineural hearing loss. Ann Otol Rhinol Laryngol. 1979;88:585–9.
2. Alexander TH, Weisman MH, Derebery JM, et al. Safety of high-dose corticosteroids for the treatment of autoimmune inner ear disease. Otol Neurotol. 2009;30:443–8.
3. Byl FM. Sudden hearing loss research clinic. Otolaryngol Clin N Am. 1978;11:71–9.
4. Moskowitz D, Lee KJ, Smith HW. Steroid use in idiopathic sudden sensorineural hearing loss. Laryngoscope. 1984;94:664–6.
5. Wilson WR, Byl FM, Laird N. The efficacy of steroids in the treatment of idiopathic sudden hearing loss. A double blind clinical study. Arch Otolaryngol. 1980;106:772–6.
6. Wilson WR. Why treat sudden hearing loss. Am J Otol. 1984;5:481–3.
7. Rauch SD. Clinical practice. Idiopathic sudden sensorineural hearing loss. N Engl J Med. 2008;359:833–40.
8. Lara Peinado A, Alcaraz Fuentes M, Plaza MG. Tratamiento sistémico corticoide en la sordera súbita idiopática. In: Plaza G, editor. Sordera súbita: diagnóstico y tratamiento. Madrid: Ergon; 2018. p. 181–90.
9. Plaza G, Durio E, Herráiz C, Asociación Madrileña de ORL, et al. Consenso sobre el diagnóstico y tratamiento de la sordera súbita. Acta Otorrinolaringol Esp. 2011;62:144–57.
10. Herrera M, García Berrocal JR, García Arumí A, et al. Update on consensus on diagnosis and treatment of idiopathic sudden sensorineural hearing loss. Acta Otorrinolaringol Esp (Engl Ed). 2019;70:290–300.
11. Stachler RJ, Chandrasekhar SS, Archer SM, American Academy of Otolaryngology-Head and Neck Surgery, et al. Clinical practice guideline: sudden hearing loss. Otolaryngol Head Neck Surg. 2012;146(Suppl. 3):S1–35.
12. Chandrasekhar SS, Tsai Do BS, Schwartz SR, et al. Clinical practice guideline: sudden hearing loss (update). Otolaryngol Head Neck Surg. 2019;161(Suppl. 1):S1–45.
13. Lawrence R, Thevasagayam R. Controversies in the management of sudden sensorineural hearing loss: an evidence-based review. Clin Otolaryngol. 2015;40:176–82.
14. Fazel MT, Jedlowski PM, Cravens RB Jr, et al. Evaluation and treatment of acute and subacute hearing loss: a review of pharmacotherapy. Pharmacotherapy. 2017;37:1600–16.
15. Murray DH, Fagan PA, Ryugo DK. Idiopathic sudden sensorineural hearing loss: a critique on corticosteroid therapy. Hear Res. 2022;422:108565.
16. Amarillo Espitia E, Bau Rodríguez P, Granda Rosales M, et al. Actitud de los otorrinolaringólogos ante la sordera súbita. In: Plaza G, editor. Sordera súbita: diagnóstico y tratamiento. Madrid: Ergon; 2018. p. 45–50.
17. Minoda R, Masuyama K, Habu K, et al. Initial steroid hormone dose in the treatment of idiopathic sudden deafness. Am J Otol. 2000;21:819–25.

18. Chen CY, Halpin C, Rauch SD. Oral steroid treatment of sudden onset sensorineural hearing loss: a ten-year retrospective analysis. Otol Neurotol. 2003;24:728–33.
19. Slattery WH, Fisher LM, Iqbal Z, et al. Oral steroid regimens for idiopathic sudden sensorineural hearing loss. Otolaryngol Head Neck Surg. 2005;132:5–10.
20. Wei B, Mubiru S, O'Leary S. Steroids for idiopathic sudden sensorineural hearing loss. Cochrane Database Syst Rev. 2006;1:CD003998.
21. Conlin AE, Parnes LS. Treatment of sudden sensorineural hearing loss: I. A systematic review. Arch Otolaryngol Head Neck Surg. 2007;133:573–81.
22. Conlin AE, Parnes LS. Treatment of sudden sensorineural hearing loss: II. A meta-analysis. Arch Otolaryngol Head Neck Surg. 2007;133:582–6.
23. Cinamon U, Bendet E, Kronenberg J. Steroids, carbogen or placebo for sudden hearing loss: a prospective double-blind study. Eur Arch Otorrinolaringol. 2001;258:477–80.
24. Song Y, Warinner CB, Suresh K, Naples JG. Roid Rage: historical perspective on the emergence of oral steroids as a treatment of idiopathic sudden sensorineural hearing loss. Otol Neurotol. 2023;44:392–7.
25. Nosrati-Zarenoe R, Hultcrantz E. Corticosteroid treatment of idiopathic sudden sensorineural hearing loss: randomized triple-blind placebo-controlled trial. Otol Neurotol. 2012;33:523–31.
26. Hultcrantz E, Nosrati-Zarenoe R. Corticosteroid treatment of idiopathic sudden sensorineural hearing loss: analysis of an RCT and material drawn from the Swedish national database. Eur Arch Otorrinolaringol. 2015;272:3169–75.
27. Wei BP, Stathopoulos D, O'Leary S. Steroids for idiopathic sudden sensorineural hearing loss. Cochrane Database Syst Rev. 2013;2013(7):CD003998.
28. Crane RA, Camilon M, Nguyen S, et al. Steroids for treatment of sudden sensorineural hearing loss: a meta-analysis of randomized controlled trials. Laryngoscope. 2015;125:209–17.
29. Maldonado Fernández M, Kornetsky S, Rubio RL. Ethics of placebo control in trials for idiopathic sudden sensorineural hearing loss. Otolaryngol Head Neck Surg. 2016;155:8–12.
30. Singh A, Kumar Irugu DV. Sudden sensorineural hearing loss—a contemporary review of management issues. J Otol. 2020;15:67–73.
31. Chen N, Karpeta N, Ma X, et al. Diagnosis, differential diagnosis, and treatment for sudden sensorineural hearing loss: current otolaryngology practices in China. Front Neurol. 2023;14:1121324.
32. Schimmer BP, Funder JW. Adrenocorticotropic hormone, adrenal steroids, and the adrenal cortex. In: Brunton LB, Hilal-Dandan R, Knollmann BC, editors. Goodman and Gilman's the pharmacological basis of therapeutics. 13th ed. New York: McGrawHill; 2018. p. 845–61.
33. Domènech Vadillo E, Merma Linares CV, Avilés Jurado FX, et al. Utilidad de los corticoides intravenosos a alta dosis en la sordera súbita idiopática. In: Plaza G, editor. Sordera súbita: diagnóstico y tratamiento. Madrid: Ergon; 2018. p. 191–6.
34. Alexiou C, Arnold W, Fauser C, et al. Sudden sensorineural hearing loss: does application of glucocorticoids make sense? Arch Otolaryngol Head Neck Surg. 2001;127:253–8.
35. Niedermeyer HP, Zahneisen G, Luppa P, Busch R, Arnold W. Cortisol levels in the human perilymph after intravenous administration of prednisolone. Audiol Neurootol. 2003;8:316–21.
36. Narozny W, Sicko Z, Przewozny T, et al. Usefulness of high doses of glucocorticoids and hyperbaric oxygen therapy in sudden sensorineural hearing loss treatment. Otol Neurotol. 2004;25:916–23.
37. Aoki D, Takegoshi H, Kikuci S. Evaluation of super-highdose steroid therapy for sudden sensorineural hearing loss. Otolaryngol Head Neck Surg. 2006;134:783–7.
38. Egli Gallo D, Khojasteh E, Gloor M, Hegemann SC. Effectiveness of systemic high-dose dexamethasone therapy for idiopathic sudden sensorineural hearing loss. Audiol Neurootol. 2013;18:161–70.
39. Raghunandhan S, Agarwal AK, Natarajan K, et al. Effect of intravenous administration of steroids in the management of sudden sensorineural hearing loss: our experience. Indian J Otolaryngol Head Neck Surg. 2013;65:229–33.
40. Gupta V, Jain A, Banerjee PK, et al. Sudden sensorineural hearing loss in adults—our experience with a multidrug high-dose steroid regimen at a tertiary care hospital. Egypt J Otolaryngol. 2016;32:105–9.

41. Song MH, Jung SY, Gu JW, Shim DB. Therapeutic efficacy of super-high-dose steroid therapy in patients with profound sudden sensorineural hearing loss: a comparison with conventional steroid therapy. Acta Otolaryngol. 2021;141:152–7.
42. Westerlaken BO, de Kleine E, van der Laan B, et al. The treatment of idiopathic sudden sensorineural hearing loss using pulse therapy: a prospective, randomized, double-blind clinical trial. Laryngoscope. 2007;117:684–90.
43. Eftekharian A, Amizadeh M. Pulse steroid therapy in idiopathic sudden sensorineural hearing loss: a randomized controlled clinical trial. Laryngoscope. 2016;126:150–5.
44. Balai E, Gupta KK, Darr A, Jindal M. Comparing the use of high dose to standard dose corticosteroids for the treatment of sudden sensorineural hearing loss in adults—a systematic review. Auris Nasus Larynx. 2024;51(1):11–24.
45. Suzuki H, Furukawa M, Kumagai M, et al. Defibrinogenation therapy for idiopathic sudden sensorineural hearing loss in comparison with high-dose steroid therapy. Acta Otolaryngol. 2003;123:46–50.
46. Suckfüll M, Plontke SK, Löhler J, et al. Idiopathic sudden sensorineural hearing loss. A clinical guideline of the German Society of Oto-Rhino-Laryngology, Head and Neck Surgery. (Updated 21/03/18). Available at : http://www.awmf.org/leitlinien/detail/ll/017-010.html (Accessed on 18 July 2022).
47. Plontke SK. Diagnostics and therapy of sudden hearing loss. GMS Curr Top Otorhinolaryngol Head Neck Surg. 2017;16:1–21.
48. Plontke SK, Girndt M, Meisner C, et al.; HODOKORT Trial Investigators. High-Dose glucocorticoids for the treatment of sudden hearing loss. NEJM Evid. 2024;3(1):EVIDoa2300172. https://doi.org/10.1056/EVIDoa2300172.
49. Kovács M, Uzsaly J, Bodzai G, et al. Efficacy of high dose systemic versus combined (systemic and intratympanic) corticosteroid therapy in idiopathic sudden sensorineural hearing loss: a prospective randomized trial and risk factor analysis. Am J Otolaryngol. 2023;45(1):104099. https://doi.org/10.1016/j.amjoto.2023.104099.
50. Koo JW, Chang MY, Yun SC, et al. The efficacy and safety of systemic injection of Ginkgo biloba extract, EGb761, in idiopathic sudden sensorineural hearing loss: a randomized placebo-controlled clinical trial. Eur Arch Otorrinolaringol. 2016;273:2433–41.
51. Yuan C, Zhang H, Sun C, Zhang K. Efficacy and safety of Ginkgo biloba extract as an adjuvant in the treatment of Chinese patients with sudden hearing loss: a meta-analysis. Pharm Biol. 2023;61:610–20.
52. Angeli SI, Abi-Hachem RN, Vivero RJ, et al. L-N-Acetylcysteine treatment is associated with improved hearing outcome in sudden idiopathic sensorineural hearing loss. Acta Otolaryngol. 2012;132:369–76.
53. Chen CH, Young YH. N-acetylcysteine as a single therapy for sudden deafness. Acta Otolaryngol. 2017;137:58–62.
54. Chen SL, Ho CY, Chin SC. Effects of oral N-acetylcysteine combined with oral prednisolone on idiopathic sudden sensorineural hearing loss. Medicine (Baltimore). 2022;101:e29792.
55. Bai X, Chen S, Xu K, et al. N-Acetylcysteine combined with dexamethasone treatment improves sudden sensorineural hearing loss and attenuates hair cell death caused by ROS stress. Front Cell Dev Biol. 2021;9:659486.
56. Bai X, Wang M, Niu X, et al. Effect of N-acetyl-cysteine treatment on sensorineural hearing loss: a meta-analysis. World J Otorhinolaryngol Head Neck Surg. 2022;8:205–12.
57. Kouka M, Bevern N, Bitter J, Guntinas-Lichius O. N-Acetylcysteine combined with prednisolone treatment shows better hearing outcome than treatment with prednisolone alone for patients with idiopathic sudden sensorineural hearing loss: a retrospective observational study. Eur Arch Otorhinolaryngol. 2024;281(1):107–16.
58. Hoes JN, Jacobs JW, Verstappen SM, et al. Adverse events of low- to medium-dose oral glucocorticoids in inflammatory diseases: a meta-analysis. Ann Rheum Dis. 2009;68:1833–8.
59. McDonough AK, Curtis JR, Saag KG. The epidemiology of glucocorticoid-associated adverse events. Curr Opin Rheumatol. 2008;20:131–7.

60. Gado M, Baschant U, Hofbauer LC, Henneicke H. Bad to the bone: the effects of therapeutic glucocorticoids on osteoblasts and osteocytes. Front Endocrinol (Lausanne). 2022;13:835720.
61. García-Berrocal JR, Ramírez-Camacho R, Lobo D, et al. Adverse effects of glucocorticoid therapy for inner ear disorders. ORL J Otorhinolaryngol Relat Spec. 2008;70:271–4.
62. Rohrmeier C, Koemm N, Babilas P, et al. Sudden sensorineural hearing loss: systemic steroid therapy and the risk of glucocorticoid-induced hyperglycemia. Eur Arch Otorrinolaringol. 2013;270:1255–61.
63. Halevy N, Elias B, Shilo S, et al. Real life safety of systemic steroids for sudden sensorineural hearing loss: a chart review. Eur Arch Otorrinolaringol. 2022;279:4787–92.
64. Toothaker RD, Craig WA, Welling PG. Effect of dose size on the pharmacokinetics of oral hydrocortisone suspension. J Pharm Sci. 1982;71:1182–5.
65. Galofré JC. Manejo de los corticoides en la práctica clínica. Rev Med Univ Navar. 2017;53:9–18.
66. Yu GH, Choi YJ, Jung HJ, et al. A comparison of single-dose and multiple divided daily-dose oral steroids for sudden sensorineural hearing loss. Braz J Otorhinolaryngol. 2019;85:733–8.
67. Weber PC. Sudden sensorineural hearing loss in adults: evaluation and management. In: Shefner JM, editor. UpToDate. Waltham, MA: UpToDate (Accessed on 11th November 2023, last update 10th May 2022).

Treatment of Idiopathic Sudden Sensorineural Hearing Loss with Intratympanic Corticosteroids

Guillermo Plaza, Mar Martínez Ruiz-Coello, Estefanía Miranda Sánchez, Cristina García García, Agustina Arbía Kalutich, Juan José Navarro Sampedro, and Concepción Rodríguez Izquierdo

Introduction

The route of administration of corticosteroids in idiopathic sudden sensorineural hearing loss (ISSNHL) has been mainly systemic: the oral route, in most cases, and the intravenous route, in certain patients with severe ISSNHL, or in countries such as Japan or Germany, whose protocols so establish [1–5]. However, some patients cannot tolerate the associated side effects of systemic corticosteroids (SCS) and at least 30–50% of patients treated with SCS do not respond to treatment and require salvage treatment.

For these reasons, the use of intratympanic corticosteroids (ITCs) has been proposed. They were first described by Silverstein et al. in 1996 [6]. The intratympanic route is a way to optimise the arrival of corticosteroids to the inner ear, while

Supplementary Information The online version contains supplementary material available at https://doi.org/10.1007/978-3-031-61385-2_8.

G. Plaza (✉)
Ear, Nose and Throat Department, Hospital Universitario de Fuenlabrada, Madrid, Spain

Ear, Nose and Throat Department, Hospital Universitario Sanitas La Zarzuela, Madrid, Spain

Universidad Rey Juan Carlos, Madrid, Spain
e-mail: guillermo.plaza@salud.madrid.org

M. Martínez Ruiz-Coello · E. Miranda Sánchez · C. García García · A. Arbía Kalutich
C. Rodríguez Izquierdo
Ear, Nose and Throat Department, Hospital Universitario de Fuenlabrada, Madrid, Spain

J. J. Navarro Sampedro
Ear, Nose and Throat Department, Hospital Universitario de Donostia, Donostia-San Sebastián, Basque Country, Spain

reducing their systemic side effects. ITCs attempt to increase the concentration and prolong the duration of the pharmacological effect of the corticosteroid on the cochlea [7]. ITCs as a treatment for ISSNHL have been used primarily as salvage treatment after SCS failure, although they may also be primary treatment as single therapy (single ITC) or in combined forms (ITC + SCS).

Pharmacodynamics: Mechanism of Action of Corticosteroids

Glucocorticoids inhibit different aspects of inflammation by stimulating or inhibiting gene transcription, and the expression of mediators, receptors, adhesion molecules and cytokines [8]. The main anti-inflammatory and immunosuppressive effect of glucocorticoids is based on the inhibition of the synthesis of numerous cytokines (IL-1, IL-2, IL-3, IL-4, IL-5, IL-6, etc.) and multiple cells (macrophages, monocytes, lymphocytes, etc.). Glucocorticoids also inhibit the effect of cytokines on target cells in different ways: on the one hand, they inhibit the synthesis of cytokine receptors; on the other hand, some cytokines produce their cellular effects by activating transcriptional factors such as AP-1 or NF-KB, the effect of which may be blocked by interaction with the receptor [7, 9].

Although the complete action of glucocorticoids within the inner ear is not well known, different local mechanisms have been demonstrated, beyond the anti-inflammatory and immunosuppressive effect, such as an increase in cochlear blood flow, a modulation in ion homeostasis, an antioxidant action, an inhibitory effect of cell apoptosis and an intense regulation of local cytokines [9–11].

There are receptors for glucocorticoids in the cochlea, with unequal expression in the different areas of it, being greater in the spiral ligament and in the vascular stria, rather than in the hair cells themselves [7].

Finally, considering that oxidative stress is one of the causes of apoptosis of hair cells, through the accumulation of ROS (reactive oxygen species) and the production of TNF-alpha, it has been described that glucocorticoids are able to reduce the expression of TNF-alpha in the spiral ligament and bind to the corticosteroid receptor to inhibit the c-Jun N-terminal kinase (JNK) pathway and activate the NF-κB signal, thus reducing oxidative stress, a pathway common to all the aetiological hypotheses of ISSNHL [7, 12].

Pharmacokinetics: Intratympanic Route into the Inner Ear

Preliminarily, in 1984, Nomura [13] demonstrated the passage of 5 mg/ml of dexamethasone injected intratympanically through the round window to the inner ear, reaching perilymphatic levels similar to those obtained after intravenous injection in guinea pigs.

Undoubtedly, the experimental studies by Parnes et al. published in 1999 have been key to understanding the pharmacokinetics of corticosteroids in the inner ear

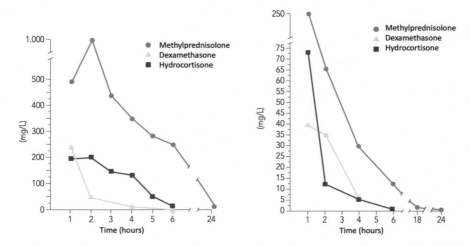

Fig. 1 Pharmacokinetics after intratympanic administration. Left: perilymph. Right: endolymph. (Modified from Parnes et al. [14]. Adapted with permission from: Parnes LS, Sun A-H, Freeman DJ. Corticosteroid pharmacokinetics in the inner ear fluids: an animal study followed by clinical application. Laryngoscope. 1999; 109(Suppl. 91): 1–17. Copyright (1999) Wiley)

[14, 15]. Using guinea pigs, they established the pharmacokinetics in the cochlear fluid for hydrocortisone, methylprednisolone and dexamethasone after oral, intravenous and intratympanic administration. They found that the three corticosteroids penetrated through the round window and reached identical levels of concentration on the vestibular and tympanic scales. In addition, the different corticosteroids had different pharmacokinetic profiles, which should be taken into account with respect to their different anti-inflammatory potency (ratio of 1/5.3 for methylprednisolone and 1/26.7 for dexamethasone, with respect to hydrocortisone).

Figure 1 shows the perilymph and endolymph concentration of the three corticosteroids after intratympanic application. The peak perilymphatic concentration is within the first and second hour, and then declines rapidly. The maximum endolymphatic peak is also between the first and second hour, and then decreases. In all samples, the concentrations reached in endolymph are higher than those reached in perilymph, which suggests the existence of an active transport that selectively concentrates the glucocorticoids within the endolymph. In this study, of the three corticosteroids analysed, methylprednisolone reached the highest corrected concentration in endolymph and perilymph, and remained for longer. Therefore, Parnes et al. concluded that methylprednisolone would be the glucocorticoid of choice for intratympanic therapy.

Similarly, the work of Chandrasekhar et al. [16, 17] found that the concentrations reached in perilymph following intratympanic application of dexamethasone were significantly higher than those obtained after intravenous administration, in guinea pigs. They also showed that there was no rise in plasma corticosteroid levels following intratympanic application.

With this contradictory evidence, there are authors who defend the intratympanic use of methylprednisolone or dexamethasone, sometimes discussing the greater effectiveness of one or the other, without a clear conclusion [7, 9].

Intratympanic Corticosteroid Administration: Recommended Method

Intratympanic drug administration is a simple procedure that only requires basic equipment in our speciality and a microscope [7, 11]. It can be done at an ENT appointment or in outpatient care. The patient should sit in a chair tilted about 45° or remain lying down, with the ear to be treated in a higher position than the contralateral.

The first step is to anaesthetise the instillation site in the tympanic membrane. Anaesthetics can be used in drops or spray with lidocaine or tetracaine (Xilonibsa®), local injection into the external auditory canal of an anaesthetic, application of EMLA (lidocaine and pilocarpine) into the canal or topical application of phenol onto the tympanic membrane. Once the area has been anaesthetised, intratympanic infiltration is performed (Fig. 2). To do this, we use a lumbar puncture needle number 22 (0.70 × 75 mm), connected to a 1 ml syringe, where we have previously loaded the corresponding medication. This type of needle can bend to facilitate access to the eardrum. Once the membrane has been perforated, we administer 0.4–0.6 ml of the drug. The appearance of bubbles while injecting is a sign that the contents are entering the middle ear. The introduction should be done slowly. It is not recommended to add lidocaine to the corticosteroid to be infiltrated.

Next, the patient must maintain the position at 45° and turn the affected ear in an upward position, avoiding swallowing and the possible tubal elimination of the drug, for about 20–30 min.

Fig. 2 Intratympanic infiltration (Illustration by Dr Sánchez). (Video present in the supplementary material, courtesy of Prof Filipo)

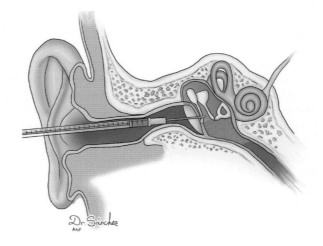

At the beginning of the treatment with ITC, some authors proposed applying it through a tympanic drainage, although this is no longer used because it can cause more residual perforations than the infiltration itself [7].

Meanwhile, in China, the subperiosteal retroauricular injection of betamethasone, instead of intratympanic infiltration, is common practice, with good results [7, 18, 19].

Posology of Intratympanic Corticosteroids

The type of glucocorticoids (methylprednisolone, dexamethasone, triamcinolone, etc.), dose, amount and frequency of ITC injections for ISSNHL depends on the authors [7, 20, 21]. Although different treatment guidelines have been published [1–5], there is no globally accepted consensus regarding the type of corticosteroid used, the route of administration or the concentration administered.

In fact, the doses vary greatly: dexamethasone, between 4 and 24 mg/ml concentration, or methylprednisolone, between 40 and 125 mg/ml, depending on each author. Similarly, dosage schedules also range from the most common, once weekly during 3 weeks, to single dose or repeat daily schedules for up to eight consecutive doses. However, no significant differences have been found between the different dosage schedules, but the treatment should start as early as possible [7, 20–24].

The ideal intratympanic application of ITC would be the one that may sustain a prolonged delivery of the drug. Since the first works by Chandrasekhar et al. [16, 17], using histamine or dimethylsulfoxide as carriers, different approaches have been tried so, for instance, through grommets, Silverstein MicroWick® or catheters [25–27]. Most have been abandoned, but some are still in use [28]. More recent approaches are based on biodegradable drug delivery implants to achieve controlled release of ITC to the inner ear [29, 30].

In the Spanish consensus [3], the administration of ITC is suggested by infiltrating a weekly dose for 3 weeks, either of methylprednisolone 0.9 cc from a 40 mg vial, or dexamethasone 0.9 cc from an 8 mg vial.

Results After Intratympanic Corticosteroids in ISSNHL

Following the landmark works of Parnes and Chandrasekhar [14–17], numerous case series, case–control studies, randomised clinical trial (RCT) and meta-analysis have been published on ITC in ISSNHL.

Probably the most important one was published in July 2022, a Cochrane review of ITC [31], based on two works by Liebau et al. [32, 33], which are very critical of all the studies published over the years.

ITC in ISSNHL as Salvage Treatment After Failure of Systemic Treatment (Salvage ITC)

Indications of Salvage ITC

In the Spanish consensus [3], treatment with ITC is recommended in cases where there is contraindication for the use of SCS or, more habitually, if there has been no response to treatment with oral or intravenous SCS within 7 days of its initiation, as rescue treatment.

In the North American consensus [5], salvage treatment with ITC is recommended in all cases where there has been no improvement after SCS between 2 and 6 weeks from the onset of symptoms.

Results of Salvage ITC

Following the work of Parnes and Chandrasekhar [14–17], numerous case series and case–control studies were published comparing salvage with ITC or not, observing better auditory results when it is used [20]. In 2004, Ho et al. [34] presented the first RCT comparing applying or not salvage ITC after failure of systemic treatment (carbogen and oral steroids) in 29 patients. Compared to not administering any ITC, applying intratympanic dexamethasone (4 mg/ml, one injection weekly, 3 weeks) achieved an improvement of >10 dB in 53% of the infiltrated patients, compared to 7% if not applied, with the mean improvement being 28 dB, compared to 13 dB if not infiltrated.

Later, different meta-analyses were able to demonstrate that ITCs, as salvage treatment after the failure of systemic treatment, are very effective, with a very favourable odds ratio (OR) [35–40]. Of note was the work published by Crane et al. [35], who found significant improvements in PTA after ITC salvage (OR 6.04; CI 3.26 vs. 11.2), while they were not found after ITC as primary treatment (OR 1.14; CI 0.82–1.59). In other words, salvage with **ITC means six times more options to obtain a hearing improvement** (Table 1).

In Spain, Plaza and Herraiz [41] published a preliminary series in 2006 of nine patients treated with salvage ITC with good results, but limited to small improvements in PTA, usually below 20 dB, as other real-life studies show [42, 43]. Furthermore, both in Denmark with the meta-analysis by Devantier et al. [44] and in Germany in a recent review of the different meta-analyses made by

Table 1 Results of ITC as ISSNHL salvage. Modified from Crane et al. [35]

	Steroids	Placebo	OR (95% CI)	Significance
Ho et al. (2004)	8/15	1/14	14.85 (1.53–144.22)	Yes
Xenellis et al. (2006)	9/19	0/18	33.47 (1.76–635.11)	Yes
Plontke et al. (2009)	6/11	5/10	1.20 (0.21–6.67)	No
Zhou et al. (2011)	17/37	8/39	3.29 (1.19–9.05)	Yes
Li et al. (2011)	9/24	0/41	50.87 (2.79–927.40)	Yes
Wu et al. (2011)	12/27	3/28	6.67 (1.61–27.52)	Yes
Total from Crane et al. (2015)			**6.04 (3.26–11.16)**	**Yes**

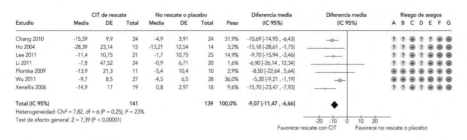

Fig. 3 Comparison of ITC versus placebo as ISSNHL salvage treatment. Mean dB improvement in PTA. Significantly favourable to salvage with ITC (mean difference −9.07; CI −11.47 to −6.66). (**a**) Selection: random sequence generation. (**b**) Selection: allocation concealment. (**c**) Performance: blinding of participants and researchers. (**d**) Detection: blinding of outcome assessor. (**e**) Attrition: incomplete outcome data. (**f**) Reporting: selective reporting. (**g**) Other biases

Estudio	CIT de rescate		No rescate o placebo		Peso	Riesgo relativo M-H, Fijo, IC 95%	Riesgo relativo M-H, Fijo, IC 95%	Riesgo de sesgos A B C D E F G
	Eventos	Total	Eventos	Total				
Ho 2004	8	15	1	14	11,2%	7,47 [1,07 , 52,33]		? ? + ? + + +
Lee 2011	10	21	4	25	39,7%	2,98 [1,09 , 8,12]		? ? + + + + +
Li 2011	9	24	0	20	5,9%	15,96 [0,99 , 258,29]		? ? + ? + + +
Plontke 2009	2	11	0	10	5,7%	4,58 [0,25 , 85,33]		+ + + + + + +
Wu 2011	12	27	3	28	32,0%	4,15 [1,31 , 13,09]		+ + + + + + +
Xenellis 2006	9	19	0	18	5,6%	18,05 [1,13 , 289,10]		? ? + ? + + +
Total (IC 95%)		117		115	100,0%	5,55 [2,89 , 10,68]		
Total de eventos:	50		8					

Heterogeneidad: Chi² = 3,08, df = 5 (P = 0,69); I² = 0%
Test de efecto general: Z = 5,14 (P < 0,00001)

0,005 0,1 1 10 200
Favorece no rescate o placebo — Favorece rescate con CIT

Fig. 4 Comparison of ITC versus placebo as ISSNHL salvage treatment. Percentage of hearing improvement. Significantly favourable to salvage with ITC (RR 5.55; CI 2.89–10.68). (**a**) Selection: random sequence generation. (**b**) Selection: allocation concealment. (**c**) Performance: blinding of participants and researchers. (**d**) Detection: blinding of outcome assessor. (**e**) Attrition: incomplete outcome data. (**f**) Reporting: selective reporting. (**g**) Other biases

Liebau et al. [32], many previous works are discussed and no such significant differences are found between the use of ITC in primary, secondary or combined form in ISSNHL. In fact, for some authors the methodology of these trials and meta-analyses has not been adequate [45].

Following the recent Cochrane meta-analysis [31], regarding ITC as salvage treatment, compared to placebo, seven studies (279 participants) were analysed. ITCs achieve a significantly greater improvement in the change in hearing threshold, although it is scarce, of about 10 dB (DM −9.07 dB better; 95% CI: −11.47 to −6.66; seven studies; 280 participants; low certainty). Salvage with ITC obtained a significantly higher difference in the proportion of participants whose hearing improved (RR 5.55; 95% CI 2.89–10.68; six studies; 232 participants; low certainty). Looking at Figs. 3 and 4, we can see that this recent meta-analysis shows a fivefold greater effect favourable towards salvage with ITC versus placebo, very similar to the meta-analysis by Crane et al. [35].

In conclusion, salvage with ITC should be performed in ISSNHL that have failed systemic treatment, even though the clinical benefit is scarce.

Salvage with ITC Versus Other Salvages

There are some studies comparing salvage treatment after systemic failure with ITC or hyperbaric oxygen therapy (HBOT). For example, Suzuki et al. [46] reviewed a series of 276 cases of ISSNHL treated with intravenous hydrocortisone (400 mg/day) and salvaged with HBOT or ITC, observing better response rates after salvage with ITC, with an OR of 2.04 in favour of ITC. In 2013, Cvoronic et al. [47] compared salvage with ITC or with HBOT in a random clinical trial on 50 patients after failure of systemic treatment. They observed that both salvages were useful and gave similar results, except in patients over 80 years for whom ITCs were more effective (40 dB vs. 21 dB improvement).

Two recent meta-analyses compared salvage after systemic failure with ITC versus HBOT. Lei et al. [48] found no differences between the two either in the proportion of patients who achieved hearing recovery, around 40–50% in both cases (RR 1.09; CI 0.83–1.42), or in the improvement of the threshold reached, around 20 dB in both cases (mean difference 0.55; CI −1.76 to 2.86). Kuo et al. [49] also did not find significant differences between the two salvages in terms of the hearing improvement obtained (improvement in PTA: 2.70; 95% CI −0.63 to 6.02). According to these studies, there seems to be no difference between salvage after systemic failure with ITC or HBOT.

ITC as Single Primary Treatment (Single ITC)

Indications of ITC as Single Primary Treatment

The Spanish consensus [3] recommends all patients diagnosed with ISSNHL be treated with corticosteroids. There are three alternatives to corticosteroid treatment, so it is up to each specialist, and depending on the patient's concomitant disease, to choose the oral route (see chapter "Treatment of Idiopathic Sudden Sensorineural Hearing Loss with Systemic Corticosteroids"), the single primary intratympanic treatment (single ITC) or combined treatment (ITC + SCS).

The North American consensus [5] considers that corticosteroids can be used as a primary treatment, not that they 'should be used' in all cases. This can be oral (SCS), ITC or ITC + SCS.

Results of ITC as Single Primary Treatment

In 2006, Kakehata et al. [50] were the first to propose the primary treatment of ISSNHL with ITC in diabetic patients. They compared the results of 21 patients treated with intravenous dexamethasone (8 mg/day, eight consecutive days) with those of 10 patients treated with intratympanic dexamethasone (4 mg/m/day, eight injections on eight consecutive days), observing a satisfactory response in 67–70% of cases, similar in both groups, but more hearing recovery after single ITC (41 dB vs. 25 dB) and fewer side effects, specifically less secondary hyperglycaemia.

In Italy, Filipo et al. [51] proposed ITC as primary treatment in a case series of 34 patients who received three infiltrations on three consecutive days with methylprednisolone (62.5 mg/ml) with a success rate of 79%. Subsequently, Filipo et al.

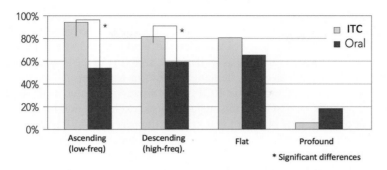

Fig. 5 Results of the clinical trial by Filipo et al. [52] comparing oral corticosteroids with intratympanic as a single primary treatment. (Courtesy of Prof. Filipo)

[52] described their results in a non-randomised clinical trial comparing SCS with single ITC. Of a total of 265 patients with ISSNHL, 48 were excluded, leaving a total of 111 who received treatment with SCS (oral prednisone for 8 days) and 106 with ITC (prednisolone one daily infiltration for three consecutive days). When comparing the results obtained, they concluded that there was no significant difference in terms of improvement in pure tone average (PTA) between both treatments (SCS vs. single ITC). However, the auditory results with single ITC were better, specifically for cases that presented losses with ascending or descending audiometric tracing (Fig. 5).

The same group of Filipo et al. [53] presented an RCT, comparing the primary treatment of ITC versus intratympanic saline solution as placebo, in a sample of 50 patients with moderate ISSNHL affecting medium frequencies. The ITC demonstrated faster and more significant improvement than the saline solution.

Labatut et al. [54] presented in 2013 the experience of the Hospital Ramón y Cajal in Madrid, Spain, with ITC as the primary treatment of ISSNHL in 35 consecutive patients (40 mg methylprednisolone, four injections in 14 days), observing complete or substantial response in 66% of patients.

Perhaps the best-known paper is the one published in 2011 by Rauch et al. [55]. This is the largest randomised clinical trial comparing the efficacy of ITC (60 mg/day prednisone, 9 days, and 5-day descending series) versus single ITC (40 mg methylprednisolone, four doses in 14 days). They included 250 patients from 16 centres, all of whom were treated within the first 14 days of SSNHL. The data did not reflect significant differences between the two types of treatments, although they were somewhat better in ISSNHL that affected low frequencies [56]. The authors concluded that the choice of one type or another of treatment should be based on medical issues associated with each patient, or in terms of medical expenses, as they are very similar.

Several systematic reviews and meta-analyses have been published on single ITC as a primary treatment for ISSNHL [21, 35, 36, 40, 57–61]. Qiang et al. [58] performed a meta-analysis including six RCTs on 225 patients treated with single ITC versus 226 patients with SS, excluding the work of Rauch et al. [55] They concluded that the group of patients treated with single ITC presented better rates of hearing recovery, as well as better results in PTA than those who received SCS. They also reviewed the heterogeneity of the analysed works regarding the hearing loss thresholds of the studied samples, as well as the variability in the treatment patterns.

Lai et al. [59] published a systematic review (in Chinese) and another meta-analysis (in English) including six RCTs of 248 patients treated with single ITC versus 236 patients with SCS. In this meta-analysis, excluding in this case the work of Filipo et al. [52], they observed that hearing improvement in PTA and recovery rate were similar in both treatments. Therefore, they recommend primary treatment with single ITC as it has fewer side effects, following the non-inferiority theses.

Finally, following the critical works of Plontke et al. [45], Liebau et al. [33] presented a detailed meta-analysis using mathematical simulations to assess the effect of ITC as a primary treatment for ISSNHL. They reviewed 25 studies conducted between 2000 and 2014, both randomised and non-randomised. They concluded that, for ITC as primary treatment, neither the drug nor the dose nor the frequency of infiltration have a prognostic influence. They rejected the use of PTA as a measure of auditory outcome because they considered that it was not appropriate, with it being better to present individual results on a case-by-case basis.

Following the recent Cochrane meta-analysis [31], regarding ITC versus SCS as a single primary treatment, they analysed 16 studies (1108 participants). ITCs achieve a significantly greater improvement in the change in hearing threshold, although it is again poor, of about 6 dB (mean difference [MD] −5.93 dB better; 95% CI: −7.61 to −4.26; 10 studies; 701 participants; low certainty). No significant difference was found in the proportion of participants whose hearing improved (RR 1.04; 95% CI: 0.97–1.12; 14 studies; 972 participants; moderate certainty). Looking at Figs. 6 and 7, we can see that the meta-analysis is somewhat favourable towards ITC versus SCS, although the conclusions of the paper do not indicate it, repeating those of the trial by Rauch et al. [55]

In conclusion, after this literature review, there seems to be no difference between treating primary cases of ISSNHL with single ITC or with SCS.

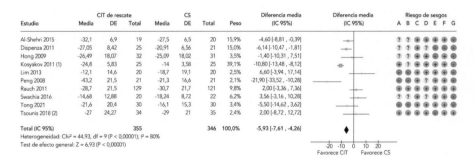

Fig. 6 Comparison of ITC versus SCS as primary treatment of ISSNHL. Mean dB improvement in PTA. Significantly favourable to ITC (mean difference −5.93; CI −7.61 to −4.26). (**a**) Selection: random sequence generation. (**b**) Selection: allocation concealment. (**c**) Performance: blinding of participants and researchers. (**d**) Detection: blinding of outcome assessor. (**e**) Attrition: incomplete outcome data. (**f**) Reporting: selective reporting. (**g**) Other biases

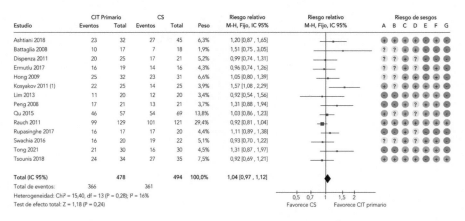

Estudio	CIT Primario Eventos	Total	CS Eventos	Total	Peso	Riesgo relativo M-H, Fijo, IC 95%	Riesgo relativo M-H, Fijo, IC 95%	A	B	C	D	E	F	G
Ashtiani 2018	23	32	27	45	6,3%	1,20 [0,87 , 1,65]								
Battaglia 2008	10	17	7	18	1,9%	1,51 [0,75 , 3,05]								
Dispenza 2011	20	25	17	21	5,2%	0,99 [0,74 , 1,31]								
Ermutlu 2017	16	19	14	16	4,3%	0,96 [0,74 , 1,26]								
Hong 2009	25	32	23	31	6,6%	1,05 [0,80 , 1,39]								
Kosyakov 2011 (1)	22	25	14	25	3,9%	1,57 [1,08 , 2,29]								
Lim 2013	11	20	12	20	3,4%	0,92 [0,54 , 1,56]								
Peng 2008	17	21	13	21	3,7%	1,31 [0,88 , 1,94]								
Qu 2015	46	57	54	69	13,8%	1,03 [0,86 , 1,23]								
Rauch 2011	99	129	101	121	29,4%	0,92 [0,81 , 1,04]								
Rupasinghe 2017	16	17	17	20	4,4%	1,11 [0,89 , 1,38]								
Swachia 2016	16	20	19	22	5,1%	0,93 [0,70 , 1,22]								
Tong 2021	21	30	16	30	4,5%	1,31 [0,87 , 1,97]								
Tsounis 2018	24	34	27	35	7,5%	0,92 [0,69 , 1,21]								
Total (IC 95%)		478		494	100,0%	1,04 [0,97 , 1,12]								
Total de eventos:	366		361											

Heterogeneidad: Chi² = 15,40, df = 13 (P = 0,28); I² = 16%
Test de efecto total: Z = 1,18 (P = 0,24)

0,5   0,7   1   1,5   2
Favorece CS   Favorece CIT primario

Fig. 7 Comparison of ITC versus SCS as primary treatment of ISSNHL. Percentage of hearing improvement. Non-significant tendency favourable to ITC (RR 1.04; CI 0.07–1.12). (**a**) Selection: random sequence generation. (**b**) Selection: allocation concealment. (**c**) Performance: blinding of participants and researchers. (**d**) Detection: blinding of outcome assessor. (**e**) Attrition: incomplete outcome data. (**f**) Reporting: selective reporting. (**g**) Other biases

ITC as Combination Treatment (ITC + SCS)

Indications
It has the same indications as ITC as a single treatment, although there are authors who recommend it when hearing loss is greater than 70 dB [21].

Results
In California, Battaglia et al. [62] were the first to present a randomised clinical trial comparing single ITC with SCS + ITC. Using oral prednisone (60 mg, maximum, followed by descending series) and/or intratympanic dexamethasone (three doses of 12 mg/ml in 3 weeks), they obtained a better and faster response with SCS + ITC, both in recovery of dB and in improvement of speech discrimination. Subsequently, these authors presented a prospective multicentre study published on 139 patients [63]. They showed that SCS+ITC (three intratympanic injections of dexamethasone, 24 mg/ml, administered weekly concomitantly with oral corticosteroid) provided a statistically significantly higher improvement in auditory parameters when compared to isolated SCS.

However, there are also publications that do not show significant differences between combination therapy versus isolated SCS. For example, Ashtiani et al. [64] published a randomised clinical trial in which 112 patients with ISSNHL were randomly divided into three groups: group 1 was administered ITC + oral placebo; group 2 was administered oral corticosteroids + intratympanic placebo and group 3 received combination therapy. In addition, all groups were given antiviral treatment and proton pump inhibitors. They concluded that there were no significant differences between the different treatments used.

Estudio	CIT Primario Eventos	CIT Primario Total	CS Eventos	CS Total	Peso	Riesgo relativo M-H, Fijo, IC 95%	Riesgo relativo M-H, Fijo, IC 95%	Riesgo de sesgos A B C D E F G
Ashtiani 2018	23	32	27	45	6,3%	1,20 [0,87 , 1,65]		
Battaglia 2008	10	17	7	18	1,9%	1,51 [0,75 , 3,05]		
Dispenza 2011	20	25	17	21	5,2%	0,99 [0,74 , 1,31]		
Ermutlu 2017	16	19	14	16	4,3%	0,96 [0,74 , 1,26]		
Hong 2009	25	32	23	31	6,6%	1,05 [0,80 , 1,39]		
Kosyakov 2011 (1)	22	25	14	25	3,9%	1,57 [1,08 , 2,29]		
Lim 2013	11	20	12	20	3,4%	0,92 [0,54 , 1,56]		
Peng 2008	17	21	13	21	3,7%	1,31 [0,88 , 1,94]		
Qu 2015	46	57	54	69	13,8%	1,03 [0,86 , 1,23]		
Rauch 2011	99	129	101	121	29,4%	0,92 [0,81 , 1,04]		
Rupasinghe 2017	16	17	17	20	4,4%	1,11 [0,89 , 1,38]		
Swachia 2016	16	20	19	22	5,1%	0,93 [0,70 , 1,22]		
Tong 2021	21	30	16	30	4,5%	1,31 [0,87 , 1,97]		
Tsounis 2018	24	34	27	35	7,5%	0,92 [0,69 , 1,21]		
Total (IC 95%)		478		494	100,0%	1,04 [0,97 , 1,12]		

Total de eventos: 366 361
Heterogeneidad: Chi² = 15,40, df = 13 (P = 0,28); I² = 16%
Test de efecto total: Z = 1,18 (P = 0,24)

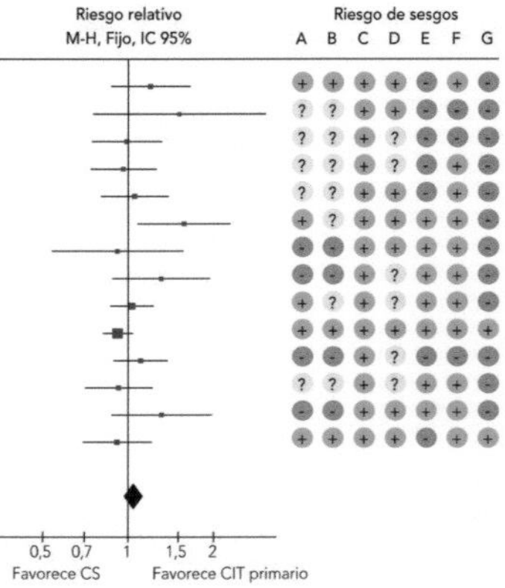

0,5 0,7 1 1,5 2
Favorece CS   Favorece CIT primario

Fig. 8 Comparison of ITC versus SCS as primary treatment of ISSNHL. Percentage of hearing improvement. Non-significant tendency favourable to ITC (RR 1.04; CI 0.07–1.12). (**a**) Selection: random sequence generation. (**b**) Selection: allocation concealment. (**c**) Performance: blinding of participants and researchers. (**d**) Detection: blinding of outcome assessor. (**e**) Attrition: incomplete outcome data. (**f**) Reporting: selective reporting. (**g**) Other biases

Systematic reviews and meta-analyses on ITC + SCS combination therapy for ISSNHL have been published [21, 65–67]. Han et al. [65] published a meta-analysis comparing combined treatment (SCS + ITC) with SCS in ISSNHL, in a group of 14 trials, with 756 patients treated with SCS +ITC and 638 with SCS. They concluded that patients treated with combination therapy had significantly better rates of hearing recovery, with an OR of 2.60 (95% CI 1.96–3.21), with more dB recovered on average and higher percentage of speech discrimination.

However, more recently, Mirian et al. [66] presented a new meta-analysis comparing SCS, single ITC and combination therapy (SCS + ITC). They included seven studies (710 patients): 325 treated with SCS, 235 with single ITC and 150 with SCS + ITC. No relevant significant differences were found between the three groups.

Following the recent Cochrane meta-analysis [31], regarding single ITC versus ITC + SCS (combination treatment) as primary treatment, 10 studies (788 participants) were identified. ITC + SCS achieve a significantly greater improvement in the change in hearing threshold, although it is again scarce, again over 8 dB (DM −8.55 dB better; 95% CI: −12.48 to −4.61; six studies; 435 participants; low certainty). A significant difference was found in the proportion of participants whose hearing improved, being greater for ITC + SCS (RR 1.27; 95% CI: 1.15–1.41; 10 studies; 788 participants; very low certainty). Looking at Figs. 8 and 9, we can see that the meta-analysis is somewhat favourable towards ITC + SCS, although the conclusions of the paper do not indicate it.

In summary, the authors of the Cochrane review are generally not in favour of ITC due to the low demonstrated effect (about 10 dB) and the lack of certainty due to the low quality of the trials. They leave the conclusions open for future studies. These studies should be more homogeneous to define improvement after treatment of ISSNHL as Osafo et al. [68] have extensively reviewed.

Estudio	Combinado: CS+CIT			CS			Peso	Diferencia media (IC 95%)	Diferencia media (IC 95%)	Riesgo de sesgos A B C D E F G
	Media	DE	Total	Media	DE	Total				
Arastou 2013	-22,6	22,2	36	-13,8	21,13	41	16,4%	-8,80 [-18,52 , 0,92]		
Arslan 2011	-21,8	18,4	58	-13	19	73	37,5%	-8,80 [-15,24 , -2,36]		
Choi 2011	-41,5	39,4	19	-33	39,4	27	2,9%	-8,50 [-31,62 , 14,62]		
Gundogan 2013	-44,05	21,53	37	-25,72	19,77	36	17,3%	-18,33 [-27,81 , -8,85]		
Lim 2013	-21,9	26,2	20	-18,7	19,1	20	7,7%	-3,20 [-17,41 , 11,01]		
Tsounis 2018	-29,8	17,71	33	-29	21	35	18,3%	-0,80 [-10,01 , 8,41]		
Total (IC 95%)			203			232	100,0%	-8,55 [-12,48 , -4,61]		

Heterogeneidad: Chi² = 7,36, df = 5 (P = 0,20); I² = 32%
Test de efecto total: Z = 4,25 (P < 0,0001)

-50   -25   0   25   50
Favorece CS+CIT   Favorece CS

Fig. 9 Comparison of single ITC versus combined ITC + SCS as primary treatment of ISSNHL. Mean dB improvement in PTA. Significantly favourable to combined treatment (mean difference −8.55; CI −12.48 to −4.61). (**a**) Selection: random sequence generation. (**b**) Selection: allocation concealment. (**c**) Performance: blinding of participants and researchers. (**d**) Detection: blinding of outcome assessor. (**e**) Attrition: incomplete outcome data. (**f**) Reporting: selective reporting. (**g**) Other biases

In conclusion, despite sometimes inconsistent results in scientific literature, there have recently been an increasing number of studies that seem to show better results of combination therapy (ITC + SCS) compared to isolated corticosteroid therapy for the treatment of SSNHL.

Complications of Intratympanic Infiltration

In general, ITC are well tolerated and have few complications. In addition, many of the complications resolve spontaneously within a few hours or days [20, 21, 69] (Table 2).

Liu et al. [70] reviewed a retrospective case series of 59 patients with ISSNHL who received a total of 278 infiltrations. They found minor complications in 1–4% of cases, including pain, tongue numbness, transient instability and tinnitus, and, to a lesser extent, major complications, such as vertigo or residual tympanic perforation. The onset of vertigo following ITC is attributed to the temperature of the instilled corticosteroid or the diffusion of lidocaine used as topical anaesthesia prior to infiltration. It is therefore recommended to warm up the corticosteroid vial for a few minutes prior to administration.

In the study by Rauch et al. [55], the group of patients treated with ITC presented instability or transient pain in 27% of cases and residual tympanic perforation in 3.8% of cases. Topf et al. [71] found 3 (1.6%) residual tympanic perforations in a series of 192 cases of ISSNHL or Ménière's disease treated with ITC. Two-thirds of patients had their eardrum closed within 1 month of the last infiltration, and the mean time to puncture closure was 18 days from the last infiltration (range 4–162 days). Hu et al. [72] evaluated 123 cases of ISNSHL treated with ITC. Also, 47% of patients had otalgia and 4% had vertigo during treatment. Meanwhile, the percentage of residual perforation was 5%.

Finally, two meta-analyses have been published on the residual perforation rate after ITC. Kim et al. [73] compared intratympanic treatment by infiltration or

Table 2 Complications of intratympanic corticosteroid treatment for ISSNHL. Modified from Vlastarakos et al. [69]

Minor complications	Treatment
Vertigo/instability	Spontaneous resolution
Nausea/vomiting	Conservative
Hearing impairment	Spontaneous resolution
Acute otitis media	Conservative
Otorrhoea	Conservative
Otalgia	Conservative
Headache	Conservative
Lingual paraesthesia	Spontaneous resolution
Dysgeusia	Spontaneous resolution
Acne	Conservative
Major complications	Treatment
Residual tympanic perforation	Myringoplasty
Chronic otitis media	Tympanoplasty

through tympanic drainage, observing a somewhat higher residual perforation rate with tympanic drainage (7.3% vs. 1.0%). However, Simani et al. [74] conducted a more recent meta-analysis, finding a similar rate of infiltration than with tympanic drainage (1.11% vs. 1.14%).

In summary, whenever an intratympanic infiltration is to be performed, the patient must be informed of these risks and sign an informed consent form, available from the Spanish Society of Otorhinolaryngology and Head & Neck Surgery (SEORL-CCC).

Conclusions

In conclusion, ITCs as primary treatment of ISSNHL are at least as effective as SCS, having the advantage of producing fewer systemic side effects than SCS and being an alternative for patients who present contraindications for systemic therapy. They are indicated as salvage of failures of systemic treatments since the probability of improving hearing is five times greater than without them.

Based on the most recent scientific evidence, combination therapy (ITC + SCS) offers better outcomes than corticosteroids in isolation in ISSNHL in terms of hearing recovery, with outcomes better in less encouraging cases such as moderate–severe hearing loss.

However, as highlighted in the recent Cochrane review on ITC [31] and expressed by some experts [75], more prospective and randomised studies with larger sample sizes and homogeneous inclusion criteria are still needed in order to obtain more conclusive results on the treatment of ISSNHL with ITC.

References

1. Rauch SD. Clinical practice. Idiopathic sudden sensorineural hearing loss. N Engl J Med. 2008;359:833–40.
2. Plaza G, Durio E, Herraiz C, Asociación Madrileña de ORL, et al. Consenso sobre el diagnóstico y tratamiento de la sordera súbita. Acta Otorrinolaringol Esp. 2011;62:144–57.
3. Herrera M, García Berrocal JR, García Arumí A, et al. Update on consensus on diagnosis and treatment of idiopathic sudden sensorineural hearing loss. Acta Otorrinolaringol Esp (Engl Ed). 2019;70:290–300.
4. Stachler RJ, Chandrasekhar SS, Archer SM, American Academy of Otolaryngology-Head and Neck Surgery, et al. Clinical practice guideline: sudden hearing loss. Otolaryngol Head Neck Surg. 2012;146(Suppl. 3):S1–35.
5. Chandrasekhar SS, Tsai Do BS, Schwartz SR, et al. Clinical practice guideline: sudden hearing loss (update). Otolaryngol Head Neck Surg. 2019;161(Suppl. 1):S1–S45.
6. Silverstein H, Choo D, Rosenberg SI, et al. Intratympanic steroid treatment of inner ear disease and tinnitus (preliminary report). Ear Nose Throat J. 1996;75:468–76.
7. Plaza MG. Tratamiento intratimpánico en la sordera súbita idiopática: Fundamentos farmacodinámicos y farmacocinéticos. In: Plaza G, editor. Sordera súbita: diagnóstico y tratamiento. Madrid: Ergon; 2018. p. 197–215.
8. Schimmer BP, Funder JW. Adrenocorticotropic hormone, adrenal steroids, and the adrenal cortex. In: Brunton LB, Hilal-Dandan R, Knollmann BC, editors. Goodman & Gilman's: the pharmacological basis of therapeutics. 13th ed. New York: McGrawHill; 2018. p. 845–61.
9. Hamid M, Trune D. Issues, indications, and controversies regarding intratympanic steroid perfusion. Curr Opin Otolaryngol Head Neck Surg. 2008;16:434–40.
10. González R, Caro J. Corticoides intratimpánicos: una revisión sistemática. Rev Otorrinolaringol Cir Cabeza Cuello. 2007;67:178–85.
11. Herraiz C, Aparicio JM, Plaza G. Intratympanic drug delivery for the treatment of inner ear diseases. Acta Otorrinolaringol Esp (Engl Ed). 2010;61:225–32.
12. Dinh CT, Goncalves S, Bas E, et al. Molecular regulation of auditory hair cell death and approaches to protect sensory receptor cells and/or stimulate repair following acoustic trauma. Front Cell Neurosci. 2015;9:96.
13. Nomura Y. Otological significance of the round window. Adv Otorhinolaryngol. 1984;33:66–72.
14. Parnes LS, Sun A-H, Freeman DJ. Corticosteroid pharmacokinetics in the inner ear fluids: an animal study followed by clinical application. Laryngoscope. 1999;109(Suppl. 91):1–17.
15. Banerjee A, Parnes LS. The biology of intratympanic drug administration and pharmacodynamics of round window drug absorption. Otolaryngol Clin North Am. 2004;37:1035–51.
16. Chandrasekhar SS, Rubinstein RY, Kwartler JA, et al. Dexamethasone pharmacokinetics in the inner ear: comparison of route of administration and use of facilitating agents. Otolaryngol Head Neck Surg. 2000;122:521–8.
17. Chandrasekhar SS. Intratympanic dexamethasone for sudden sensorineural hearing loss: clinical and laboratory evaluation. Otol Neurotol. 2001;22:18–23.
18. Lv L, Gao Z, Liu J, et al. Comparison between postauricular steroid injection and intratympanic steroid perfusion for refractory severe and profound sudden sensorineural hearing loss. Am J Otolaryngol. 2022;43:103189.
19. Li Y, Liang J, Chiang HJ, et al. Postauricular injection in the treatment of all-frequency and high frequency descending sudden hearing loss: a protocol for systematic review and meta-analysis. Medicine (Baltimore). 2021;100:e23847.
20. Amarillo Espitia E, Plaza MG. Tratamiento intratimpánico en la sordera súbita idiopática como rescate tras fracaso del tratamiento sistémico. In: Plaza G, editor. Sordera súbita: diagnóstico y tratamiento. Madrid: Ergon; 2018. p. 217–30.
21. Pasamontes Pingarrón JA, Plaza MG. Tratamiento intratimpánico en la sordera súbita idiopática como tratamiento primario único o combinado. In: Plaza G, editor. Sordera súbita: diagnóstico y tratamiento. Madrid: Ergon; 2018. p. 231–43.

22. Sáenz-Piñones JC, Villarreal IM, García-Chilleron R, et al. Intratympanic methylpredniso-lone for sudden sensorineural hearing loss: comprehensive reexamination of the model. J Otolaryngol ENT Res. 2015;3:251–7.
23. Nelson L, Swanson D, Borowiec E, et al. The impact of intratympanic steroid dosage on hearing recovery in sudden sensorineural hearing loss. Ann Otol Rhinol Laryngol. 2023;132:879–87.
24. Wang Y, Gao G, Wang L, et al. Association between the number of intratympanic steroid injec-tions and hearing recovery in sudden sensorineural hearing loss. Front Neurol. 2021;12:798569.
25. Silverstein H, Thompson J, Rosenberg SI, Brown N, Light J. Silverstein MicroWick. Otolaryngol Clin North Am. 2004;37:1019–34.
26. Plontke SK, Löwenheim H, Mertens J, et al. Randomized, double blind, placebo controlled trial on the safety and efficacy of continuous intratympanic dexamethasone delivered via a round window catheter for severe to profound sudden idiopathic sensorineural hearing loss after failure of systemic therapy. Laryngoscope. 2009;119:359–69.
27. Salt AN, Plontke SK. Principles of local drug delivery to the inner ear. Audiol Neurootol. 2009;14:350–60.
28. Moreno I, Belinchon A. Evaluating the efficacy of intratympanic dexamethasone in protecting against irreversible hearing loss in patients on cisplatin-based cancer treatment: a randomized controlled phase IIIB clinical trial. Ear Hear. 2022;43:676–84.
29. Plontke SK, Liebau A, Lehner E, et al. Safety and audiological outcome in a case series of ter-tiary therapy of sudden hearing loss with a biodegradable drug delivery implant for controlled release of dexamethasone to the inner ear. Front Neurosci. 2022;16:892777.
30. Lei X, Yin X, Hu L, et al. Delivery of dexamethasone to the round window niche by satu-rated gelatin sponge for refractory sudden sensorineural hearing loss: a preliminary study. Otol Neurotol. 2023;44:e63–7.
31. Plontke SK, Meisner C, Agrawal S, et al. Intratympanic corticosteroids for sudden sensorineu-ral hearing loss. Cochrane Database Syst Rev. 2022;7:CD008080.
32. Liebau A, Pogorzelski O, Salt AN, et al. Hearing changes after intratympanic steroids for sec-ondary (salvage) therapy of sudden hearing loss: a meta-analysis using mathematical simula-tions of drug delivery protocols. Otol Neurotol. 2018;39:803–15.
33. Liebau A, Pogorzelski O, Salt AN, et al. Hearing changes after intratympanically applied ste-roids for primary therapy of sudden hearing loss: a meta-analysis using mathematical simula-tions of drug delivery protocols. Otol Neurotol. 2017;38:19–30.
34. Ho HG, Lin HC, Shu MT, et al. Effectiveness of intratympanic dexamethasone injection in sudden-deafness patients as salvage treatment. Laryngoscope. 2004;114:1184–9. Frequently misquoted as Guan-Min et al
35. Crane RA, Camilon M, Nguyen S, et al. Steroids for treatment of sudden sensorineural hearing loss: a meta-analysis of randomized controlled trials. Laryngoscope. 2015;125:209–17.
36. Garavello W, Galluzzi F, Gaini RM, et al. Intratympanic steroid treatment for sudden deafness: a meta-analysis of randomized controlled trials. Otol Neurotol. 2012;33:724–9.
37. Li H, Feng G, Wang H, et al. Intratympanic steroid therapy as a salvage treatment for sudden sensorineural hearing loss after failure of conventional therapy: a meta-analysis of random-ized, controlled trials. Clin Ther. 2015;37:178–87.
38. Ng JH, Ho RC, Cheong CS, et al. Intratympanic steroids as a salvage treatment for sudden sensorineural hearing loss? A meta-analysis. Eur Arch Otorhinolaryngol. 2015;272:2777–82.
39. Barreto MA, Ledesma AL, de Oliveira CA, et al. Intratympanic corticosteroid for sudden hear-ing loss: does it really work? Braz J Otorhinolaryngol. 2016;82:353–64.
40. El Sabbagh NG, Sewitch MJ, Bezdjian A, et al. Intratympanic dexamethasone in sudden sen-sorineural hearing loss: a systematic review and meta-analysis: Intratympanic dexamethasone for SSHL. Laryngoscope. 2017;127:1897–908.
41. Plaza G, Herráiz C. Intratympanic steroids for treatment of sudden hearing loss after failure of intravenous therapy. Otolaryngol Head Neck Surg. 2007;137:74–8.
42. Ringrose T, Biggs TC, Jones L, et al. Salvage intratympanic steroid therapy for sudden sensori-neural hearing loss: our real-life experience in 32 patients. J Laryngol Otol. 2022;136:827–30.

43. Li LQ, Bennett AMD. Probability of clinically significant hearing recovery following salvage intratympanic steroids for sudden sensorineural hearing loss in the 'real world'. J Laryngol Otol. 2022;136:831–8.
44. Devantier L, Callesen HE, Jensen LR, et al. Intratympanic corticosteroid as salvage therapy in treatment of idiopathic sudden sensorineural hearing loss: a systematic review and meta-analysis. Heliyon. 2022;8:e08955.
45. Plontke SK. Diagnostics and therapy of sudden hearing loss. GMS Curr Top Otorhinolaryngol Head Neck Surg. 2017;16:1–21.
46. Suzuki H, Hashida K, Nguyen KH, et al. Efficacy of intratympanic steroid administration on idiopathic sudden sensorineural hearing loss in comparison with hyperbaric oxygen therapy. Laryngoscope. 2012;122:1154–7.
47. Cvorovic L, Jovanovic MB, Milutinovic Z, et al. Randomized prospective trial of hyperbaric oxygen therapy and intratympanic steroid injection as salvage treatment of sudden sensorineural hearing loss. Otol Neurotol. 2013;34:1021–6.
48. Lei X, Feng Y, Xia L, et al. Hyperbaric oxygen therapy versus intratympanic steroid for salvage treatment of sudden sensorineural hearing loss: a systematic review and meta-analysis. Otol Neurotol. 2021;42:e980–6.
49. Kuo TC, Chao WC, Yang CH, et al. Intratympanic steroid injection versus hyperbaric oxygen therapy in refractory sudden sensorineural hearing loss: a meta-analysis. Eur Arch Otorhinolaryngol. 2022;279:83–90.
50. Kakehata S, Sasaki A, Oji K, et al. Comparison of intratympanic and intravenous dexamethasone treatment on sudden sensorineural hearing loss with diabetes. Otol Neurotol. 2006;27:604–8.
51. Filipo R, Covelli E, Balsamo G, et al. Intratympanic prednisolone therapy for sudden sensorineural hearing loss: a new protocol. Acta Otolaryngol. 2010;130:1209–13.
52. Filipo R, Attanasio G, Russo FY, et al. Oral versus short-term intratympanic prednisolone therapy idiopathic sudden hearing loss. Audiol Neurootol. 2014;19:225–33.
53. Filipo R, Attanasio G, Russo FY, et al. Intratympanic steroid therapy in moderate sudden hearing loss: a randomized, triple-blind, placebo-controlled trial. Laryngoscope. 2013;123:774–8.
54. Labatut T, Daza MJ, Alonso A. Intratympanic steroids as primary initial treatment of idiopathic sudden sensorineural hearing loss. The Hospital Universitario Ramón y Cajal experience and review of the literature. Eur Arch Otorhinolaryngol. 2013;270:2823–32.
55. Rauch SD, Halpin CF, Antonelli PJ, et al. Oral vs intratympanic corticosteroid therapy for idiopathic sudden sensorineural hearing loss: a randomized trial. JAMA. 2011;305:2071–9.
56. Halpin C, Rauch SD. Using audiometric thresholds and word recognition in a treatment study. Otol Neurotol. 2006;27:110–6.
57. O'Connell BP, Hunter JB, Haynes DS. Current concepts in the management of idiopathic sudden sensorineural hearing loss. Curr Opin Otolaryngol Head Neck Surg. 2016;24:413–9.
58. Qiang Q, Wu X, Yang T, et al. A comparison between systemic and intratympanic steroid therapies as initial therapy for idiopathic sudden sensorineural hearing loss: a meta-analysis. Acta Otolaryngol. 2017;137:598–605.
59. Lai D, Zhao F, Jalal N, et al. Intratympanic glucocorticosteroid therapy for idiopathic sudden hearing loss: meta-analysis of randomized controlled trials. Medicine (Baltimore). 2017;96:e8955.
60. Yang T, Liu H, Chen F, et al. Intratympanic vs systemic use of steroids as first-line treatment for sudden hearing loss: a meta-analysis of randomized, controlled trials. J Otol. 2021;16:165–77.
61. Mirsalehi M, Ghajarzadeh M, Farhadi M, et al. Intratympanic corticosteroid injection as a first-line treatment of the patients with idiopathic sudden sensorineural hearing loss compared to systemic steroid: a systematic review and meta-analysis. Am J Otolaryngol. 2022;43:103505.
62. Battaglia A, Burchette R, Cueva R. Combination therapy (intratympanic dexamethasone + high-dose prednisone taper) for the treatment of idiopathic sudden sensorineural hearing loss. Otol Neurotol. 2008;29:453–60.

63. Battaglia A, Lualhati A, Lin H, et al. A prospective multi-centered study of the treatment of idiopathic sudden sensorineural hearing loss with combination therapy versus high-dose prednisone alone: a 139 patient follow-up. Otol Neurotol. 2014;35:1091–8.

64. Ashtiani MK, Firouzi F, Bastaninejad S, et al. Efficacy of systemic and intratympanic corticosteroid combination therapy vs intratympanic or systemic therapy in patients with idiopathic sudden sensorineural hearing loss: a randomized controlled trial. Eur Arch Otorhinolaryngol. 2018;275:89–97.

65. Han X, Yin X, Du X, et al. Combined intratympanic and systemic use of steroids as a first-line treatment for sudden sensorineural hearing loss: A meta-analysis of randomized, controlled trials. Otol Neurotol. 2017;38:487–95.

66. Mirian C, Ovesen T. Intratympanic vs systemic corticosteroids in first-line treatment of idiopathic sudden sensorineural hearing loss: a systematic review and meta-analysis. JAMA Otolaryngol Head Neck Surg. 2020;146:421–8.

67. Sialakis C, Iliadis C, Frantzana A, et al. Intratympanic versus systemic steroid therapy for idiopathic sudden hearing loss: a systematic review and meta-analysis. Cureus. 2022;14:e22887.

68. Osafo NK, Friedland DR, Harris MS, et al. Standardization of outcome measures for intratympanic steroid treatment for idiopathic sudden sensorineural hearing loss. Otol Neurotol. 2022;43:1137–43.

69. Vlastarakos PV, Papacharalampous G, Maragoudakis P, et al. Are intra-tympanically administered steroids effective in patients with sudden deafness? Implications for current clinical practice. Eur Arch Otorhinolaryngol. 2012;269:363–80.

70. Liu YC, Chi FH, Yang TH, et al. Assessment of complications due to intratympanic injections. World J Otorhinolaryngol Head Neck Surg. 2016;2:13–6.

71. Topf MC, Hsu DW, Adams DR, et al. Rate of tympanic membrane perforation after intratympanic steroid injection. Am J Otolaryngol. 2017;38(1):21–5.

72. Hu CY, Lien KH, Chen SL, et al. Complications and prognosis associated with intra-tympanic steroid injection to treat sudden sensorineural hearing impairment. Am J Otolaryngol. 2022;43:103221.

73. Kim YH, Lee DY, Lee DH, et al. Tympanic membrane perforation after intratympanic steroid injection: a systematic review and meta-analysis. Otolaryngol Head Neck Surg. 2022;166:249–59.

74. Simani L, Shilo S, Oron Y, et al. Residual perforation risk assessment of intratympanic steroids via tympanostomy tube versus transtympanic injections. Laryngoscope. 2021;131:E2583–91.

75. Murray DH, Fagan PA, Ryugo DK. Idiopathic sudden sensorineural hearing loss: a critique on corticosteroid therapy. Hear Res. 2022;422:108565.

Treatment of Idiopathic Sudden Sensorineural Hearing Loss with Hyperbaric Oxygen Therapy

Ana María García Arumí, Jordi Desola Alà, Paula López Mesa, and María Pujol Rodríguez

Introduction

Hyperbaric oxygen therapy (HBOT) is based on 100% oxygen respiration within a chamber at a pressure several times higher than atmospheric pressure. Its immediate result is an increase in partial oxygen pressure (PaO$_2$) and a logarithmic increase in plasma oxygen. This allows for greater cell exchange by capillarity and simple gradient oxygen diffusion, even in areas compromised by ischaemic, toxic or metabolic hypoxia, to which conventional drugs do not have access. At the same time, hyperoxia promotes an exuberant formation of physiological antioxidants that counteract the possible occurrence of toxic effects [1].

The therapeutic application of HBOT extends to chronic soft-tissue infections, radio-induced lesions of bone, muscle and mucous membranes, and necrotising soft-tissue infections. In the field of emergencies, in addition to its fundamental indication in dysbaric accidents, HBOT makes it possible to treat acute carbon monoxide and hydrocyanic monoxide poisoning, central retinal artery occlusions and idiopathic sudden sensorineural hearing loss (ISSNHL) without known cause.

In ISSNHL, HBOT acts as a biological treatment to restore cellular homeostasis and enhance natural mechanisms of spontaneous recovery thanks to the decrease in

A. M. García Arumí (✉)
Ear, Nose and Throat Department, Hospital Vall d'Hebron, Barcelona, Spain

Faculty of Medicine and Psychology, Universidad Autónoma de Barcelona, Barcelona, Spain

J. Desola Alà
Centro de Recuperación e Investigaciones Submarinas—Unidad de Terapia Hiperbárica (CRIS-UTH) [Centre for Underwater Recovery and Research—Hyperbaric Therapy Unit], Hospital Moisès Broggi, Sant Joan Despí, Barcelona, Spain

Hyperbaric Medicine at the Universidad de Barcelona, Barcelona, Spain

P. López Mesa · M. Pujol Rodríguez
Ear, Nose and Throat Department, Hospital Vall d'Hebron, Barcelona, Spain

G. Plaza, J. R. García Berrocal (eds.), *Sudden Sensorineural Hearing Loss*, https://doi.org/10.1007/978-3-031-61385-2_9

inflammatory response and the major increase in the supply of dissolved plasma oxygen that easily accesses the terminal circulation [2, 3]. In these cases, the optimisation of HBOT calls for the elimination of coincident pharmacological treatments that may interfere with the spontaneous normalisation process.

Rationale for HBOT Treatment for ISSNHL

To date, several hypotheses have been suggested on the most important mechanisms for the onset of ISSNHL. The most important factor is thought to be ischaemia due to reduced blood flow to the inner ear.

The cochlea and its structures, particularly the vascular stria and the organ of Corti, require a high supply of oxygen. However, direct vascular input, particularly to the organ of Corti, is minimal [4]. Tissue oxygenation occurs through the oxygen diffusion from the cochlear capillary networks in the perilymph and the cortilymph. Perilymph is the main source of oxygen for intracochlear structures, and when its partial oxygen pressure decreases to 70%, intracochlear oxygenation cannot continue auditory function [5].

HBOT is the only known method to significantly increase O_2 in inner ear fluids. HBOT maximises the partial pressure of oxygen delivered to the inner ear, reduces the ischaemic effect [6] and stimulates the cellular metabolism of the inner ear, even when blood supply is insufficient [7].

Several studies, including systematic reviews and meta-analyses, have shown that HBOT as a combination treatment with corticosteroid therapy for ISSNHL is superior to isolated corticosteroid therapy. This is true both as an initial and as a salvage option [8–13] as long as the treatment schedule, treatment pressure and hyperbaric device used are correct. The final result will be conditioned to the delay in the start of HBOT application.

In 2016, the tenth European Consensus Conference of the European Committee for Hyperbaric Medicine (ECHM) recommended HBOT for the treatment of ISSNHL (type 1 recommendation, level B evidence), according to which HBOT is recommended as a consolidated therapy in many studies, publications and consolidated experiences [2, 13].

In the update of the American Academy of Otolaryngology-Head and Neck Surgery's Clinical Practice Guidelines on ISSNHL, the association of HBOT to corticosteroid treatment was proposed as an initial optional treatment, in the first 2 weeks, or salvage, within 1 month, from the onset of symptoms [14]. Similarly, in the current Spanish consensus on SSNHL, it is also recommended as salvage treatment.

Indications of HBOT Treatment for ISSNHL

Treatment guidelines for all indications, safety recommendations and accident prevention methods are regulated by specialised international societies: the ECHM in Europe and the Undersea & Hyperbaric Medical Society (UHMS) in the United States. Both institutions play an important quality control role in the correct and safe application of HBOT. The European Code of Good Practice for Hyperbaric Medicine and other European regulations govern the use of hyperbaric chambers, either monoplace (for a single patient) or multiplace for several patients simultaneously with surveillance and medical assistance inside the chamber during treatment (Figs. 1 and 2).

The ECHM, after its Multidisciplinary Consensus Conference, held in Lille (France) in 2016, recommends treatment batches of no less than 15 sessions in the acute phase, at a pressure between 2 and 2.5 absolute atmosphere (ATA). Depending on the results obtained, and in cases of clear progressive improvement, the treatment plan may be prolonged at the discretion of the specialists in charge [2, 15]. Regrettably, however, some private business-oriented institutions and companies do not respect these agreed European guidelines and apply empirical approaches based on individual observations. It is very important to prioritise and limit the selection of indications to healthcare establishments that follow the guidelines established by the ECHM and its related committees.

The ENT Department of the Vall d'Hebron University Hospital collaborates with CRIS-UTH, the hyperbaric therapy unit of Barcelona, located in the Moisès Broggi Hospital in Sant Joan Despí, which strictly follows the recommendations of the ECHM in terms of therapeutic guidelines, safety systems and accident prevention.

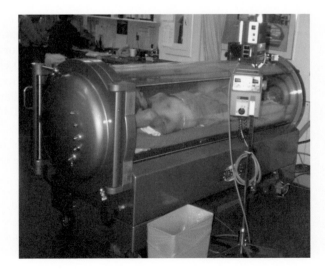

Fig. 1 Well-equipped monoplace hyperbaric chamber located at Moisés Broggi Hospital, Sant Joan Despí, Barcelona

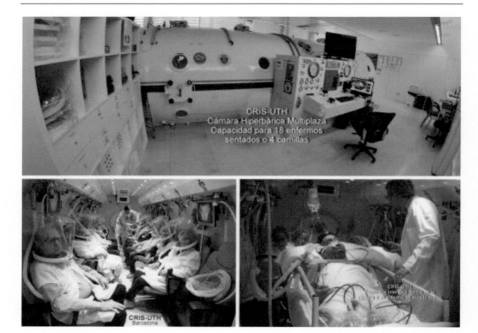

Fig. 2 CRIS-UTH multiplace chamber located at Moisés Broggi Hospital, Sant Joan Despí, Barcelona

Importance of Delayed Initiation of HBOT Treatment

In the literature, special attention is paid to the time elapsed between the onset of symptoms and the start of treatment for ISSNHL, with emphasis on the need for rapid initiation. Most studies, methodologically correct, have shown that early initiation of HBOT is more effective than a late onset [8, 16, 17]. The most favourable prognoses refer to patients with medium or profound hearing loss, for whom HBOT was implemented within the first few days of the onset of hearing loss symptoms.

In the CRIS-UTH experience, with more than 400 cases of ISSNHL treated, there was a significant improvement in 68% of patients received up to 4 weeks after the debut of sudden hearing loss. However, only patients who received HBOT within the first 5 days after hearing loss experienced full improvement with total recovery from hearing [18].

Complications of HBOT Treatment

If ECHM and/or UHMS recommendations are followed, HBOT application is safe and with few side effects [1, 15, 19, 20].

The most common side effect of HBOT, which can occur at a frequency of 8.9–66.7%, is middle ear barotrauma. However, although their observation is always linked to a technical or methodological defect in the application of HBOT, patients must learn to use the well-known Valsalva or Toynbee manoeuvres, swallowing or moving the jaw from side to side, with which the possibility of a middle ear barotrauma is low. The possibility of barotrauma is much greater when a small volume monoplace chamber is used in which pressure changes are more abrupt and patients cannot be cared for during treatment.

Less frequent is sinus barotrauma which, if detected early, forces the discontinuation of treatment as there is no procedure to neutralise it once established.

In long-term treatments for more than 40 sessions, 20% of patients may suffer from so-called hyperbaric myopia. This is a transient disorder that spontaneously reverses between 1 and 2 months after the end of treatment [19]. HBOT, when applied in monoplace chambers pressurised with pure oxygen, can accelerate the evolution of cataracts after 35 sessions. It can also occur in monoplace chambers in which whole oxygenation hood is used. However, if the guideline established by the ECHM is applied, the possibility of both ophthalmic side effects is null [2].

Patients with a history of spontaneous pneumothorax should be carefully evaluated by the medical team before starting treatment as a possible contraindication. Claustrophobia will be an exclusion criterion for treatment in small-volume hyperbaric chambers and in all monoplace chambers. In larger multiplace chambers, most of these patients are able to adapt thanks to the care of the specialised health team that accompanies them during treatment.

Advantages and Disadvantages of HBOT Treatment for ISSNHL

The evolution of hearing recovery in ISSNHL is unpredictable as the underlying pathogenesis is variable. There are many factors related to prognosis (age, degree of hearing loss, type of audiogram, start of treatment, associated conditions, etc.). Because approximately one- to two-thirds of patients can recover spontaneously within 1 week of the onset of the condition, it is difficult to determine which patients should receive steroid treatment, as well as the dose and start time, given their side effects.

While most patients with mild hearing loss recover, the group of patients with severe hearing loss, and especially those with contralateral hearing loss and for whom treatment with steroids is not effective, pose a greater challenge for finding more conclusive alternatives. The efficacy of HBOT as a salvage treatment for patients refractory to corticosteroid therapy is widely established in several controlled studies [9, 12, 21–23].

The only limitation in the application of HBOT is the availability of referring these patients to specialised centres and the application of the appropriate procedure [2, 15]. However, currently hyperbaric medicine centres exist with multiplace or monoplace chambers of proven quality and efficacy. In addition to Sant Joan Despí, Barcelona, there are centres in the Spanish cities of Santander, Palamós, Castellón, Alicante, Cartagena, Málaga, Cádiz, Vigo, Ferrol, Madrid, Zaragoza, Palma de Mallorca, Menorca and Ibiza. Although outside Spain, the hyperbaric centres in

Perpignan (France), Lisbon and Porto (Portugal) should also be considered due to their proximity.

For obvious reasons of safety and efficacy, referral to public or private centres using low-pressure devices and/or not applying high oxygen concentrations should be avoided. The treatment pressure should always be at least two absolute atmosphere and the oxygen concentration 100%. Oxygen tents with internal oxygen concentration devices that slightly increase the atmospheric pressure as a side effect should also be avoided as they cannot be classified as hyperbaric or even low-pressure chambers.

To better validate the beneficial effects of HBOT treatment for ISSNHL, randomised comparative studies of the effects on auditory recovery in ISSNHL with HBOT as the initial treatment option against corticosteroids would be necessary, in addition to those already performed as salvage treatment [24–26]. While the latest Cochrane review [27] concludes that there is no evidence of steroid efficacy in ISSNHL, this is currently the most universal treatment, as endorsed by recent meta-analyses [9–12]. For this reason, the design of a comparative study between hyperbaric treatment alone without corticosteroids, compared to conventional steroid therapy, should not present an ethical problem.

The global experience in treating ISSNHL with HBOT is currently very high. Among hyperbaric specialists around the world there is the presumption, and in many cases the conviction, that outcomes are more favourable in patients who have received HBOT alone without the addition of other medications, than when applied in combination with steroids. This is due to the well-known anti-regenerative capacity of steroids over many structures, and to the side effects and long-term effects thereof, which discourage their indiscriminate use [11, 28]. Therefore, it would be justified and very interesting to carry out a two-arm design, always initiating both treatments in the first few days of hearing loss.

Conclusions

The result of combined corticosteroid and HBOT treatment for ISSNHL shows an increase in hearing improvement. The sooner treatment with HBOT is started, the better the prognosis. When hyperbaric treatment is initiated immediately, it is possible to obtain a complete recovery of hearing function.

It is necessary to always apply the guideline recommended by the ECHM, as well as respect safety and accident prevention procedures.

It is convenient as well to assess the likely greater effect of HBOT if applied alone, without addition of drugs or other treatments.

References

1. Desola J. Indicaciones actuales de la Oxigenoterapia hiperbárica. Formación Médica Continuada en Atención Primaria. FMC. 2009;16:507–23.

2. Desola J. Oxigenoterapia hiperbárica en el siglo XXI. Análisis crítico y reflexiones. Formación Médica Continuada en Atención Primaria. FMC. 2017;24:116–33.
3. Liu XH, Liang F, Jia XY, et al. Hyperbaric oxygen treatment improves hearing level via attenuating TLR4/NF-kappaB mediated inflammation in sudden sensorineural hearing loss patients. Biomed Environ Sci. 2020;33:331–7.
4. Nagahara K, Fisch U, Yagi N. Perilymph oxygenation in sudden and progressive sensorineural hearing loss. Acta Otolaryngol. 1983;96:57–68.
5. Lamm H, Klimpel L. Hyperbaric oxygen therapy in internal ear and vestibular disorders. Preliminary report. HNO. 1971;19:363–9.
6. Goto F, Fujita T, Kitani Y, et al. Hyperbaric oxygen and stellate ganglion blocks for idiopathic sudden hearing loss. Acta Otolaryngol. 1979;88:335–42.
7. Fattori B, Berrettini S, Casani A, et al. Sudden hypoacusis treated with hyperbaric oxygen therapy: a controlled study. Ear Nose Throat J. 2001;80:655–60.
8. Capuano L, Cavaliere M, Parente G, et al. Hyperbaric oxygen for idiopathic sudden hearing loss: is the routine application helpful? Acta Otolaryngol. 2015;135:692–7.
9. Rhee TM, Hwang D, Lee JS, et al. Addition of hyperbaric oxygen therapy vs medical therapy alone for idiopathic sudden sensorineural hearing loss: a systematic review and meta-analysis. JAMA Otolaryngol Head Neck Surg. 2018;144:1153–61.
10. Bayoumy AB, Lammet van der Veen E, Alexander de Ru J. Hyperbaric oxygen therapy vs medical therapy for sudden sensorineural hearing loss. JAMA Otolaryngol Head Neck Surg. 2019;145:699–700.
11. Ahn Y, Seo YJ, Lee YS. The effectiveness of hyperbaric oxygen therapy in severe idiopathic sudden sensorineural hearing loss. J Int Adv Otol. 2021;17:215–20.
12. Joshua TG, Ayub A, Wijesinghe P, et al. Hyperbaric oxygen therapy for patients with sudden sensorineural hearing loss: a systematic review and meta-analysis. JAMA Otolaryngol Head Neck Surg. 2022;148:5–11.
13. Mathieu D, Marroni A, Kot J. Tenth European Consensus Conference on Hyperbaric Medicine: recommendations for accepted and non-accepted clinical indications and practice of hyperbaric oxygen treatment. Diving Hyperb Med. 2017;47:24–32.
14. Chandrasekhar SS, Tsai Do BS, Schwartz SR, et al. Clinical practice guideline: sudden hearing loss (update). Otolaryngol Head Neck Surg. 2019;161(Suppl. 1):S1–45.
15. García Arumí AM, Mateo Monfort A, Desola AJ. Tratamiento con oxigenoterapia hiperbárica en la sordera súbita idiopática. In: Plaza G, editor. Sordera súbita: diagnóstico y tratamiento. Madrid: Ergon; 2018. p. 249–58.
16. Xie S, Qiang Q, Mei L, et al. Multivariate analysis of prognostic factors for idiopathic sudden sensorineural hearing loss treated with adjuvant hyperbaric oxygen therapy. Eur Arch Otorrinolaringol. 2018;275:47–51.
17. Wang Y, Gao Y, Wang B, et al. Efficacy and prognostic factors of combined hyperbaric oxygen therapy in patients with idiopathic sudden sensorineural hearing loss. Am J Audiol. 2019;15(28):95–100.
18. Desola J, Gómez M, Papoutsidakis E, et al. Treatment of sudden deafness with hyperbaric oxygen. A descriptive analysis of 190 cases. In: ICHM-2014. XIXth International Congress on Hyperbaric Medicine. Cape Town, South Africa. [Downloaded from https://www.cris-uth.cat/investigacion/ on 10 April 2022].
19. Desola J. Contraindicaciones y Efectos secundarios de la Oxignoterapia hiperbárica. [Downloaded from https://www.cris-uth.cat/asistencia/contraindicaciones-efectos-secundarios/ on 10 April 2022].
20. Kim H, Kong SK, Kim J, et al. The optimized protocol of hyperbaric oxygen therapy for sudden sensorineural hearing loss. Laryngoscope. 2023;133:383–8.
21. Huang C, Tan G, Xiao J, et al. Efficacy of hyperbaric oxygen on idiopathic sudden sensorineural hearing loss and its correlation with treatment course: prospective clinical research. Audiol Neurootol. 2021;26:479–86.

22. Tong B, Niu K, Ku W, et al. Comparison of therapeutic results with/without additional hyperbaric oxygen therapy in idiopathic sudden sensorineural hearing loss: a randomized prospective study. Audiol Neurootol. 2021;26:11–6.
23. Bagli BS. Clinical efficacy of hyperbaric oxygen therapy on idiopathic sudden sensorineural hearing loss. Undersea Hyperb Med. 2020;47:51–6.
24. Cvorovic L, Jovanovic MB, Milutinovic Z, et al. Randomized prospective trial of hyperbaric oxygen therapy and intratympanic steroid injection as salvage treatment of sudden sensorineural hearing loss. Otol Neurotol. 2013;34:1021–6.
25. Kuo TC, Chao WC, Yang CH, et al. Intratympanic steroid injection versus hyperbaric oxygen therapy in refractory sudden sensorineural hearing loss: a meta-analysis. Eur Arch Otorrinolaringol. 2022;279:83–90.
26. Lei X, Feng Y, Xia L, et al. Hyperbaric oxygen therapy versus intratympanic steroid for salvage treatment of sudden sensorineural hearing loss: a systematic review and meta-analysis. Otol Neurotol. 2021;42:e980–6.
27. Wei BP, Stathopoulos D, O'Leary S. Steroids for idiopathic sudden sensorineural hearing loss. Cochrane Database Syst Rev. 2013;7:CD003998.
28. Moody-Antonio SA, Chandrasekhar SS, Derebery MJ. Is it time to encourage hyperbaric oxygen therapy in combination with medical treatment for sudden sensorineural hearing loss? JAMA Otolaryngol Head Neck Surg. 2022;148:11–2.

Single-Sided Deafness (SSD) Hearing Aids: Airway Hearing Aids, Bone Conduction Hearing Aids and Cochlear Implant Electrical Stimulation

Ignacio Pla Gil, María Aragonés Redó,
Tomàs Pérez Carbonell, and Jaime Marco Algarra

Introduction

In this chapter, we will describe the different treatment options for patients with unilateral (cophotic) severe-profound sensorineural hearing loss with normal contralateral hearing, also known as single-sided deafness (SSD) [1–3]. SSD is estimated to affect between 12 and 27 people per 100,000 inhabitants of the general population. Most SSD cases that appear abruptly in adults are after a case of idiopathic sudden sensorineural hearing loss (ISSNHL) that has not improved [4], highlighting the consequences of having monaural hearing.

Characteristics of Monaural Hearing

People with binaural hearing enjoy certain advantages [5]. The primary advantage is a better signal-to-noise ratio (SNR), which improves intelligibility in noisy environments. The second results from the binaural processing of the signal by the brain, which is able to separate noise and speech from different places, using the inter-aural differences of time, signal and spectral levels, thereby tuning intelligibility. A third advantage is related to the binaural redundancy effect, responsible for improved speech perception through the identification of identical signals reaching both ears.

I. Pla Gil (✉) · M. Aragonés Redó · T. Pérez Carbonell
Ear, Nose and Throat Department, Hospital Clínic Universitari de València, Valencia, Spain

J. Marco Algarra
Ear, Nose and Throat Department, Hospital Clínic Universitari de València, Valencia, Spain

Universidad de Valencia, Valencia, Spain

However, a patient with SSD has difficulty locating sound sources, worse intelligibility when the signal comes to the side with hearing loss due to the head shadow effect, poor intelligibility in background noise environments (especially when the noise comes from the side of the healthy ear) and loss of the redundancy effect of binaurality (summation) [1, 3, 4].

As far as localisation is concerned, we are able to localise sound thanks to the ability to detect interaural differences in the time, intensity and phase of sound between the two ears. In the case of SSD, this ability is lost because the comparison between both ears is not possible. The head shadow effect, first described by Tillman et al. [6], assumes that the intensity of a sound is attenuated from one side of the head to the other, averaging 6.4 dB SPL when it reaches the contralateral ear [7]. In addition, this attenuation depends on frequency, so the higher the sound, the more attenuation. This can directly affect intelligibility, making it worse.

Regarding poor intelligibility in background noise environments, many authors have published the advantages of binaural hearing to reduce the harmful effect of noise (squelch) or reverberation for correct intelligibility. Gulick et al. [8] observed an improvement in intelligibility when there was binaural hearing versus monaural hearing, being the basis of central auditory processing and giving rise to different auditory information on each side that helped separate sounds into auditory components. The same author also described the summation effect of binaurality with respect to monaurality, as an advantage in the processing of information, specifically in the detection of thresholds. Thus, if both ears are audiologically symmetrical, the threshold is approximately 3 dB better than the monaural threshold. This difference increases to 6 dB with supra-threshold stimuli, which implies a direct effect on the improvement of intelligibility.

In addition to all these hearing difficulties, the patient may suffer from early listening fatigue in conversations due to excessive attention. The appearance of psychological effects, such as stress or a feeling of isolation or social exclusion, also determines that a treatment option should be taken into account to try to reduce the difficulties described. Another factor to consider is that SSD is generally accompanied by a certain degree of tinnitus as more than 90% of adults who experience unilateral sensorineural hearing loss also suffer from it [8].

Treatment of Single-Sided Deafness (SSD)

The ideal objective would be the total rehabilitation of binaurality, which would lead to the disappearance of all the problems generated by monaural hearing. A cochlear implant (CI) is the only device capable of directly stimulating the cophotic ear. However, it is more common to use hearing aids on the healthy ear: auditory osseointegrated devices (AOD) and devices with contralateral routing of signal (CROS) and BiCROS technology.

Hearing Aids for SSD

Types of Hearing Aids for the Treatment of SSD

It is important that the candidate knows and understands the audiological expectations of their treatment, but equally important is that the otolaryngologist knows the patient's needs before choosing the most suitable hearing aid.

The presence of unilateral severe-profound sensorineural hearing loss means that this ear will not benefit from the adaptation of a conventional auditory prosthesis due to the poor intelligibility and possible hearing loss caused by the major amplification [7, 9].

Different research projects have shown that these patients do benefit from a variety of hearing-enhancing devices. The foundation, in general, is to stimulate the healthy ear from the reception of sound in the ear with hearing loss, eliminating the head shadow effect. The transmission of sound from the affected ear to the healthy ear will vary depending on the type of device, dividing the mechanisms of action into three groups.

Bone Hearing Aids for SSD

These are devices similar to conventional auditory prostheses that are adapted bilaterally. They have been in use for four decades. The hearing aid of the cophotic ear only acts as a receiver and transmitter of sound, and its function is to receive the sound and transport it to the auditory prosthesis that is in the healthy ear (via a cable or via wireless systems). The hearing aid of the healthy ear may or may not amplify the signal [10]. There are two systems: CROS and BiCROS.

1. CROS (contralateral routing of signal). The microphone of the hearing aid located in the 'bad' ear picks up the sound coming from that side of the head and sends it to the hearing aid receiver of the 'good' ear so that it can hear it, without amplifying the sound (Fig. 1).
2. BiCROS (bilateral contralateral routing of signal). The microphone of the hearing aid located in the 'bad' ear picks up the sound coming from that side of the head and sends it to the hearing aid of the 'good' ear. Since the 'good' ear has a certain degree of hearing loss, the second microphone of the hearing aid receiver picks up the sound of the 'good' ear and amplifies all sounds so that the user can hear them more effectively (Fig. 2).

Bone Conduction Hearing Implants

Implants designed for bone conduction (Fig. 3) include auditory osseointegrated devices (AODs), active AODs (Bonebridge™, Ossia®), SoundBite®, TransEar®, Transcranial CROS, etc.

1. AODs (auditory osseointegrated devices): Currently the most used option by otolaryngologists in the treatment of SSD, thanks to their good performance and results, as well as involving a well-tolerated and non-complex surgical technique

Fig. 1 Image showing the operation of CROS devices

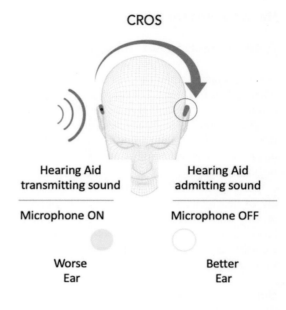

Fig. 2 Image showing the operation of BiCROS devices

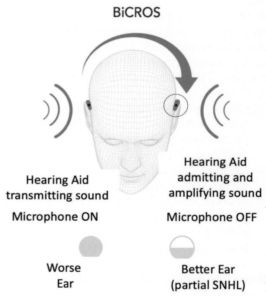

[11]. AODs can be divided into two major groups according to the publications made by Reinfeldt et al. [12]: direct conduction, which in turn are divided into percutaneous and active transcutaneous; and skin conduction, also known as passive AODs.

Fig. 3 Classification of bone-conduction hearing aids

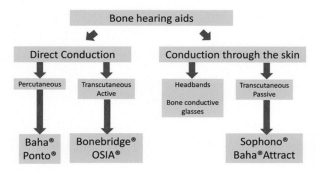

Fig. 4 Percutaneous bone hearing aids

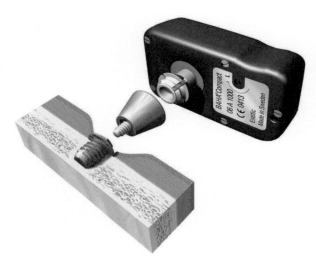

The device that fits into the cophotic ear acts as the receiver of the signal. Unlike CROS, these do act as emitters and only one device is needed. The signal produced is transported by bone conduction to the healthy contralateral ear, which stimulates it.

There are different anchoring mechanisms: percutaneous and transcutaneous. When the healthy ear has thresholds <20 dB, both systems will give good results [13] (Fig. 4).

2. Cochlear Osia®: In recent years, a new active transcutaneous bone conduction system has emerged, known as Cochlear Osia® (Fig. 5). It offers the advantages of active transcutaneous implants, such as fewer skin complications and better aesthetics, and, in addition, thanks to the transduction of sound through a piezo-electric material, it is able to generate greater output power compared to current percutaneous systems.

A recent study by Pla-Gil et al. [14] in moderate-grade mixed hearing loss patients showed that this new device is capable of producing a tonal improve-

Fig. 5 Cochlear Osia
device

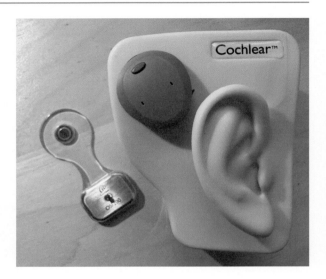

Fig. 6 SoundBite device

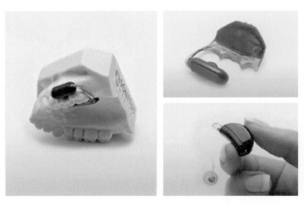

ment in the free field at medium and high frequencies, as well as an improvement
in silent and noise intelligibility.

3. TransEar®: In terms of aesthetics, this is similar to a conventional hearing aid;
   the difference is that instead of having a speaker to amplify the sound, it includes
   an oscillator that is placed in contact with the bone portion of the EAC of the
   cophotic ear so that it uses transcranial bone conduction to stimulate the contralateral cochlea. These devices should not be used in case of narrow EAC or ears
   with chronic otorrhea [15].

4. SoundBite™: A receiver hearing aid is placed in the cophotic ear, processing the
   sound signal, transforming it and wirelessly sending it to the device that will be
   placed at the level of the molars in the upper dental arch on the same side as the
   healthy ear. This intraoral device produces the mechanical signal by stimulating
   the cochlea [16] (Fig. 6).

Indications for Hearing Aids in SSD

According to the recommendations of audiological guides, the ideal candidate with SSD would have tonal thresholds in the frequencies 500, 1000, 2000 and 3000 Hz $\leq$ 20 dB via air (VA), in the best ear ('healthy ear') [17]. In clinical practice, the indication can be extended to subjects suffering from mild–moderate hearing loss in the healthy ear with current AODs and BiCROS systems [18].

Therefore, any patient with SSD with normal hearing could benefit from the whole range of devices mentioned above depending on the choice of one or another of the factors indicated below:

- Anatomical contraindications: Such as edentulous patients, in the case of SoundBite®; very narrow atresias or external auditory canals (EACs) that make it impossible to adapt a CROS, BiCROS or TransEar® system; in the case of AODs, insufficient skull thickness for correct osseointegration; or when a CI is chosen, problems with internal ear malformation or retrocochlear pathology.
- Audiometric parameters: Audiometric thresholds should be used as a starting point for the choice of one device or another. However, we should not only be guided by this, as thresholds will not predict results [19].
- Transcranial attenuation (TA): This should be evaluated in each candidate to adapt the AOD. Studies show that there is great variability in TA between subjects, although they conclude that TA < 10 dB can be a good predictor of performance.
- Trial period: Many studies recommend this as it provides a real and highly predictive experience of the results. However, there is no consensus on the duration and it is not clear whether this test influences the choice of one device or another. It should be conducted whenever possible, but there are devices where this test cannot be offered (TransEAR®, transcranial CROS or SoundBite®).
- Intelligibility with background noise: Poor or insufficient intelligibility is one of the main reasons for the patient to decline adaptation of the device. Therefore, it would be advisable to perform speech audiometry exams with background noise.
- Subjective measures: Questionnaires that assess the benefit, handicap reduction, location, etc., can help in the choice of the device. Examples would be the Bern Benefit in Single-Sided Deafness, Abbreviated Profile of Hearing Aid Benefit (APHAB) and Speech Spatial Qualities (SSQ) questionnaires.
- In addition, the selection of one device or another will also depend on aesthetic criteria, the refusal to undergo surgery and peculiarities of the device such as technical characteristics, ease of use, healthy ear occlusion, cost and social security coverage.

Assessment of the Candidate for a Hearing Aid for SSD

Candidate

It is important to present the different options available, explain the advantages and disadvantages and advise on the best option for their case.

When evaluating a candidate for rehabilitative treatment with hearing aids, measures that distinguish the degree of disability and in such a way as to delimit a reference point for future outcome evaluations should be incorporated. Therefore, the objectives would be, firstly, to quantify hearing loss based on audiological studies and, secondly, to qualify the associated disability, as well as the subjective assessment.

As additional considerations, hearing monitoring should be included, at least up to 1 year, to ensure that hearing loss is stable before any invasive intervention is performed.

Audiological Assessment

This is an ophthalmic examination (including a thorough physical examination and CT and/or MRI, if applicable) and a complete audiological study:

- Pure tone audiometry (PTA) ISO 8253-1.2010: airway (AW), bone pathway (BP) and calculation of transcranial attenuation, if required.
- Transcranial attenuation should be measured in each of the patients in whom AOD treatment is being considered. The measurement will be taken when calculating the difference between the BP threshold in the good ear and the BP threshold at the site where the final AOD would be implanted. The use of a more powerful device is recommended in order to ensure greater signal power that compensates for the attenuating effect offered by the skin and headset.
- Silent speech audiometry (SA) (ISO 8253-3, 2012): Calculating the speech recognition threshold (SRT) and the percentage of discrimination (%D).
- VA with background noise: It is preferable to perform this in order to predict the performance of the devices and the elimination of the head shadow effect.

We recommend setting the VA with the signal (list of two-syllable words) at 45° or 90° next to the ear with hearing loss and noise at 45° or 90° on the side of the best ear [20, 21].

Likewise, Van de Heyning et al. [22] published in 2016 a consensus for the study of SSD, including VA in different configurations for the study of the benefits of binaurality (head shadow effect, binaural redundancy effect and squelch effect), sound source location tests and quality-of-life questionnaires. The objective was to establish a protocol that would compare the results and better record the advantages and disadvantages in the different treatment options of SSD.

Patient Perception, Communication Needs and Selection of Treatment Goals

Apart from the audiological assessment, the communication difficulties identified by the patient should be examined and used to identify the treatment goals. After obtaining this information, the choice of the hearing aid that meets these characteristics can be discussed with more realistic expectations.

Our recommendation is that each patient should be evaluated with validated questionnaires before a hearing aid is selected in order to provide more realistic expectations of its use.

Today, there are numerous questionnaires that measure different variables related to hearing aids and implants. The most cited is the Nijmegen Cochlear Implant Questionnaire (NCIQ), validated in Spanish. This is a quality-of-life questionnaire that assesses the changes perceived by the patient with regard to hearing, language and other psychosocial aspects. This has the advantage of assessing the subjective situation of the patient before and after receiving their device or implant.

Trial Period

The home trial period of AODs should be reserved for patients who meet the audiological requirements.

In the case of AODs, for patients who preferably have a transcranial attenuation ≤10 dB and who, after testing with the device, have observed an audiological improvement.

Preferably, the device provided should be the most efficient available and should have previously been adjusted to the individual requirements of each user.

Results of Hearing Aids for SSD

The older CROS models consisted of two analogue hearing aids connected together by a cable along the neck. Users reported poor aesthetic acceptance, discomfort from healthy ear occlusion and poor sound quality related to distortion. In addition, they reported the ineffective reduction of ambient noise, electromagnetic interference with other devices and the possible worsening of the intelligibility of the healthy ear due to the signal coming from the cophotic ear. All these facts meant that users or ENT specialists themselves did not choose this technology. A similar situation happened with old AODs, with patients referring to poor sound quality and little benefit.

In recent years, both CROS hearing aids and AODs have undergone a substantial improvement with new models, with aesthetic and technological improvements, digital sound, signal processing strategies that improve their quality or the use of wireless transmission. All these advances have made both technologies seriously viable for the treatment of SSD and, in our field, AODs are the best treatment option.

Regarding the difficulties that accompany SSD, several studies have found that both CROS and AODs do not show an improvement in sound localisation [23, 24]. With regard to the perception of speech with background noise compared to performance without hearing aids, there are several advantages and disadvantages that CROS systems and AODs can cause. As a main advantage, although both devices cannot restore binaural hearing, they are effective in reducing the head shadow effect and, therefore, can improve speech perception, especially when speech originates on the cophotic side. However, as a disadvantage, these devices could hinder performance in cases where speech is on the healthy side and noise on the affected side, transmitting noise to the healthy side [1].

AODs and CROS devices are equipped with noise reduction circuits and directional microphones. As advantages of AODs over CROS, Flynn et al. [25] published an improvement in noise management when the direction of the noise source was on the cophotic side. The benefits of directional microphones in AODs have been investigated, but few on CROS devices exist.

With regard to subjective measures, there are numerous publications on them and most advocate a greater perception of auditory benefit and satisfaction with AODs than with CROS systems. Better performance with AODs is also objective in noise conditions [1].

Cochlear Implants for SSD

The audiological results obtained with CROS and AODs do not fully meet the expectations of some patients and do not fully restore binaurality. Although they are effective in addressing the head shadow effect, they do not provide psychoacoustic information to the deaf side (binaural suppression effect and summation effect), so they fail to help improve speech perception in noise [2].

Based on these facts, the use of rehabilitation methods that could restore bilateral auditory input could lead to an improvement in spatial hearing and speech perception in patients with SSD. If the ideal objective is the total rehabilitation of binaurality, the use of CI makes sense and, although its indication is not currently widespread, there are several articles on this concept.

Usefulness of Cochlear Implants for SSD

The indication of CI in SSD is recent [26, 27]. In fact, there is a concern about the brain's ability to distinguish between acoustic and electrical stimuli, and also the doubt that CI hearing interferes with the processing of the acoustic signal of the good ear.

However, a CI is the only option that provides information to the cophotic ear and therefore would potentially benefit binaural listening in patients with SDD. In addition, noise recognition and sound localisation are superior in binaural hearing [28].

To date, general selection criteria for cochlear implantation for SSD have not yet been established and factors that may affect outcomes are unknown. However, we are seeing that as familiarity with CI increases, there is a broadening of the selection criteria for surgery.

Results of CI for SSD

Regarding studies in terms of sound localisation, several studies showed that sound localisation is better with the use of CI than in conditions without help or with CROS systems or with AODs, presenting statistically significant differences [29–32].

Implanted ear intelligibility, when assessed in silent conditions, has been shown to improve significantly after implantation. However, when understanding is measured with background noise, the results are highly variable and the parameters differ considerably between researchers, making comparison difficult. Several studies describe an improvement in intelligibility with background noise. However, only four have shown consistent statistical data [29, 30, 33, 34]. All four used different audiometric tests to measure the result. Two of the studies found a significant improvement in speech comprehension when sound is emitted to the cochlear-implanted side and noise to the ear with normal hearing, considered the most challenging situation in everyday life. Only Távora-Vieira et al. [34] found a statistically superior performance when the signal and noise were emitted from the same source versus the subject, 0° azimuth (S_0/N_0). The above-mentioned results are encouraging as they could be attributed to the fact that the auditory system can process binaural signals and restore the binaural suppression effect after cochlear implantation thanks to central auditory processing, resulting in different acoustic information on each side and helping to separate sounds into auditory components.

CI was first used in 2008 to treat tinnitus in patients with SSD and may now be the new indication for CI that has created the most consensus [35]. Several studies confirm the favourable effect of CI in the treatment of tinnitus, when retraining therapy, sound therapy and drugs have not been effective. Tinnitus improvement may occur due to various mechanisms such as habituation, sound masking, direct stimulation of the cochlear nerve or reorganisation of the cortical pathways. Among the studies that evaluated the relief or suppression of tinnitus perception, several presented statistically significant reductions of the symptom [34–36]. This improvement in tinnitus perception after cochlear implantation supports the theory of auditory deafferentation, resulting from the restoration of auditory input through an acoustic stimulus.

In a recent meta-analysis analysing only case series, Blasco and Redleaf [37] found that CIs had a statistically significant improvement in tinnitus severity. Van Zon et al. [38] analysed six studies and reported a significant reduction in tinnitus distress in three of them.

Meanwhile, the duration of hearing loss is a well-known factor that affects hearing performance in post-lingual patients undergoing CI [39]. In 2015, Távora-Vieira et al. [34] were the first to investigate whether hearing loss duration and age at implantation have an effect on outcomes in post-lingual patients with SSD. The study showed that these variables do not appear to affect speech perception with background noise or tinnitus improvement. In addition, their results suggest that patients with SSD may be able to integrate acoustic and electrical signals. This concept has not been studied extensively and is still controversial due to concerns about the brain's ability to integrate acoustic-electrical stimuli and the fear that CI interferes with the acoustic signal processing of the good ear.

However, there is a high degree of heterogeneity between the results and the different studies [40–44], as well as in the selection of patients in terms of duration and time of onset of hearing loss. In addition, the studies differ in follow-up and, especially, in the tests and parameters used to evaluate the results [32]. These differences largely prevent a direct comparison between the studies.

Experience at Valencia University Hospital with CI for SSD

To date, we have 9 patients with SSD using implants and 11 patients with asymmetric hearing loss using implants, with a follow-up that in some cases reaches 4 years. Below are the results of the SSD group. We have observed a subjective improvement in the Nijmegen Questionnaire in all subscales, with the subscales of basic and advanced perception of sound and in social activities and interactions being statistically significant. In addition, with regard to intelligibility with background noise, we emitted speech audiometry exams with different signal-to-noise ratios (SNR −3; 0 and +10 dB) and speakers placed at 0° and 90° (in the ear to be implanted or already implanted), varying the way of emitting both the signal (S) and the masking noise (N). In our study we observed that, as the signal on noise increases, as is logical, the percentages of intelligibility increase.

The use of CI increases intelligibility in all situations, except in the worst possible situation (SNR-3) in which it remains without showing statistically significant differences. In the S0°R0° and SicR0° situations with both 0 dB SNR and + 10 dB SNR, a statistically significant improvement was shown with the use of the cochlear implant. Finally, we can see an improvement in the perception of tinnitus with the use of CI after comparing the scores obtained with the Tinnitus Handicap Index (THI), with statistically significant improvements in both the total score and in the emotional, functional and catastrophic components.

Conclusions

When there is no improvement after sudden hearing loss and the ear is cophotic, single-sided deafness (SSD) occurs, which we must try to rehabilitate. It is important that the candidate knows and understands the audiological expectations of their treatment, but equally important is that the otolaryngologist knows the patient's needs before choosing the hearing aid.

The audiological results obtained with the current auditory osseointegrated devices (AODs) and Contralateral Routing of Signal (CROS) technology, although they improve the head shadow effect, are not so ambitious as to provide an improvement in speech perception or localisation.

The ideal goal will be the total rehabilitation of binaurality through the rehabilitation of the cophotic ear with a cochlear implant (CI). However, there is major clinical heterogeneity between studies evaluating cochlear implantation in patients with SSD. The results regarding the improvement of sound localisation, intelligibility and, mainly, tinnitus improvement, are promising indications. However, quality studies and evidence are required before CI is standardised as treatment for SSD. Since CI appears to provide greater benefits than CROS systems and AODs, it could become the first treatment option for patients with short-term SSD.

References

1. Pla Gil I, García Callejo FJ, Redondo Martínez J, et al. Dispositivos auditivos para el tratamiento del oído único (Single-Sided Deafness). In: Plaza G, editor. Sordera súbita: diagnóstico y tratamiento. Madrid: Ergon; 2018. p. 271–6.
2. Pla Gil I, Martínez Benyto P, Morant Ventura A, et al. Implante coclear en la sordera neurosensorial unilateral. In: Plaza G, editor. Sordera súbita: diagnóstico y tratamiento. Madrid: Ergon; 2018. p. 277–81.
3. Linstrom CJ, Silverman CA, Yu GP. Efficacy of the bone anchored hearing aid for single sided deafness. Laryngoscope. 2009;119:713–20.
4. Usami SI, Kitoh R, Moteki H, et al. Etiology of single-sided deafness and asymmetrical hearing loss. Acta Otolaryngol. 2017;137(Suppl. 565):S2–7.
5. Vermeire K, Van de Heyning P. Binaural hearing after cochlear implantation in subjects with unilateral sensorineural deafness and tinnitus. Audiol Neurootol. 2009;14:163–71.
6. Tillman T, Kasten R, Horner I. Effect of head shadow on reception of speech. ASHA. 1963;5:778–9.
7. Lekue A, Lassaleta L, Gavilán J. Evaluación auditiva del oído único. In: Manrique Rodríguez M, Marco Algarra J, editors. Audiología. Ponencia Oficial de la Sociedad Española de Otorrinolaringología y Patología Cérvico-Facial 2014. Madrid: CYAN, Proyectos Editoriales, SA; 2014. p. 295–304.
8. Gulick WL, Gescheider GA, Frisina RD. Hearing: physiological acoustics, neural coding, and psychoacoustics. New York: Oxford University Press; 1989. ISBN 0–19–504307-3
9. Carreño F, García V, Valverde J. Audífonos y generadores de ruido. In: Manrique Rodríguez M, Marco Algarra J, editors. Audiología. Ponencia Oficial de la Sociedad Española de Otorrinolaringología y Patología Cérvico-Facial 2014. Madrid: CYAN, Proyectos Editoriales, SA; 2014. p. 307–22.
10. Bishop CE, Eby TL. The current status of audiologic rehabilitation for profound unilateral sensorineural hearing loss. Laryngoscope. 2010;120:552–6.
11. Gavilan J, Adunka O, Agrawal S, et al. Quality standards for bone conduction implants. Acta Otolaryngol. 2015;135:1277–85.
12. Reinfeldt S, Håkansson B, Taghavi H, et al. New developments in bone-conduction hearing implants: a review. Med Devices (Auckl). 2015;8:79–93.
13. Dumper J, Hodgetts B, Liu R, et al. Indications for bone-anchored hearing aids: a functional outcomes study. J Otolaryngol Head Neck Surg. 2009;38:96–105.
14. Pla-Gil I, Redó MA, Pérez-Carbonell T, et al. Clinical performance assessment of a new active osseointegrated implant system in mixed hearing loss: results from a prospective clinical investigation. Otol Neurotol. 2021;42:e905–10.
15. Battista RA, Mullins K, Wiet RM, et al. Sound localization in unilateral deafness with the Baha or TransEar device. JAMA Otolaryngol Head Neck Surg. 2013;139:64–70.

16. Gurgel RK, Shelton C. The SoundBite hearing system: patient-assessed safety and benefit study. Laryngoscope. 2013;123:2807–12.
17. Martín L, de Valmaseda MJ, Cavalle Garrido L, Huarte Irujo A, et al. Clinical guideline on bone conduction implants. Acta Otorrinolaringol Esp (Engl Ed). 2019;70:105–11.
18. Kinkel M. Cutting the wire part II: fitting wireless CROS/BiCROS devices in practice. Available at: http://www.audiologyonline.com/articles/cutting-wire-part-ii-fitting-767.
19. Desmet J, Bouzegta R, Hofkens A, et al. Clinical need for a Baha trial in patients with single-sided sensorineural deafness. Analysis of a Baha database of 196 patients. Eur Arch Otorrinolaringol. 2012;269:799–805.
20. Snapp HA, Fabry DA, Telischi FF, et al. A clinical protocol for predicting outcomes with an implantable prosthetic device (BAHA) in patients with single-sided deafness. J Am Acad Audiol. 2010;21:654–62.
21. Stenfelt S. Bilateral fitting of BAHAs and BAHA® fitted in unilateral deaf persons: acoustical aspects. Int J Audiol. 2005;44:178–89.
22. Van de Heyning P, Távora-Vieira D, Mertens G, et al. Towards a unified testing framework for single-sided deafness studies: a consensus paper. Audiol Neurootol. 2016;21:391–8.
23. Baguley D, Bird J, Humphriss R, et al. The evidence base for the application of contralateral bone anchored hearing aids in acquired unilateral sensorineural hearing loss in adults. Clin Otolaryngol. 2006;31:6–14.
24. Hol MK, Kunst SJ, Snik AF, et al. Pilot study on the effectiveness of the conventional CROS, the transcranial CROS and the BAHA transcranial CROS in adults with unilateral inner ear deafness. Eur Arch Otorhinolaryngol. 2010;267:889–96.
25. Flynn MC, Hedin A, Halvarsson G, et al. Hearing performance benefits of a programmable power BAHA® sound processor with a directional microphone for patients with a mixed hearing loss. Clin Exp Otorhinolaryngol. 2012;5(Suppl. 1):S76–81.
26. Kamal SM, Robinson AD, Diaz RC. Cochlear implantation in single-sided deafness for enhancement of sound localization and speech perception. Curr Opin Otolaryngol Head Neck Surg. 2012;20:393–7.
27. Manrique M, Ramos Á, de Paula VC, et al. Guía clínica sobre implantes cocleares. Acta Otorrinolaringol Esp. 2019;70:47–54.
28. Offeciers E, Morera C, Müller J, et al. International consensus on bilateral cochlear implants and bimodal stimulation. Acta Otolaryngol. 2005;125(9):918–9.
29. Arndt S, Aschendorff A, Laszig R, et al. Comparison of pseudobinaural hearing to real binaural hearing rehabilitation after cochlear implantation in patients with unilateral deafness and tinnitus. Otol Neurotol. 2011;32:39–47.
30. Firszt JB, Holden LK, Reeder RM, et al. Cochlear implantation in adults with asymmetric hearing loss. Ear Hear. 2012;33:521–33.
31. Cardieux JH, Firszt JB, Reeder RM. Cochlear implantation in nontraditional candidates: preliminary results in adolescents with asymmetric hearing loss. Otol Neurotol. 2013;34:408–15.
32. Härkönen K, Kivekäs I, Rautiainen M, et al. Single-sided deafness: the effect of cochlear implantation on quality of life, quality of hearing, and working performance. ORL J Otorhinolaryngol Relat Spec. 2015;77:339–45.
33. Vermeire K, Nobbe A, Schleich P, et al. Neural tonotopy in cochlear implants: an evaluation in unilateral cochlear implant patients with unilateral deafness and tinnitus. Hear Res. 2008;245:98–106.
34. Távora-Vieira D, Marino R, Acharya A, et al. The impact of cochlear implantation on speech understanding, subjective hearing performance, and tinnitus perception in patients with unilateral severe to profound hearing loss. Otol Neurotol. 2015;36:430–6.
35. Van de Heyning P, Vermeire K, Diebl M, et al. Incapacitating unilateral tinnitus in single-sided deafness treated by cochlear implantation. Annals Otol Rhinol Laryngol. 2008;117:645–52.
36. Mertens G, Kleine Punte A, De Ridder D, et al. Tinnitus in a single-sided deaf ear reduces speech reception in the nontinnitus ear. Otol Neurotol. 2013;34:662–6.

37. Blasco MA, Redleaf MI. Cochlear implantation in unilateral sudden deafness improves tinnitus and speech comprehension: meta-analysis and systematic review. Otol Neurotol. 2014;35:1426–32.
38. van Zon A, Peters JP, Stegeman I, et al. Cochlear implantation for patients with single-sided deafness or asymmetrical hearing loss: a systematic review of the evidence. Otol Neurotol. 2015;36:209–19.
39. Blamey P, Artieres F, Başkent D, et al. Factors affecting auditory performance of postlinguistically deaf adults using cochlear implants: an update with 2251 patients. Audiol Neurootol. 2013;18:36–47.
40. Buss E, Dillon MT, Rooth MA, et al. Effects of cochlear implantation on binaural hearing in adults with unilateral hearing loss. Trends Hear. 2018;22:1–15.
41. Falcón Benítez N, Falcón González JC, Ramos Macías Á, et al. Cochlear implants in single-sided deafness. comparison between children and adult populations with post-lingually acquired severe to profound hearing loss. Front Neurol. 2021;12:760831.
42. Deep NL, Spitzer ER, Shapiro WH, et al. Cochlear implantation in adults with single-sided deafness: outcomes and device use. Otol Neurotol. 2021;42:414–23.
43. Ludwig AA, Meuret S, Battmer RD, et al. Sound localization in single-sided deaf participants provided with a cochlear implant. Front Psychol. 2021;12:753339.
44. Rader T, Waleka OJ, Strieth S, et al. Hearing rehabilitation for unilateral deafness using a cochlear implant: the influence of the subjective duration of deafness on speech intelligibility. Eur Arch Otorrinolaringol. 2023;280:651–9.

Future Perspectives in Idiopathic Sudden Sensorineural Hearing Loss

Guillermo Plaza, Juan José Navarro Sampedro,
Carlos O'Connor Reina, Concepción Rodríguez Izquierdo,
and José Ramón García Berrocal

Introduction

Medicine is a science in constant evolution and full of uncertainty. As William Osler said: 'The greater the ignorance, the greater the dogmatism'. This is especially true for diseases little known as idiopathic sudden sensorineural hearing loss (ISSNHL), and about which there is much therapeutic controversy and few robust studies [1–5].

Currently, there are three lines of research that will bring new therapies into ISSNHL. First, new drugs whose design is aimed at the pathophysiological bases of cochlear oxidative stress. Second, new pharmacokinetics are designed to increase diffusion and prolong the time of action of drugs that are used intratympanically.

G. Plaza (✉)
Ear, Nose and Throat Department, Hospital Universitario de Fuenlabrada, Madrid, Spain

Ear, Nose and Throat Department, Hospital Universitario Sanitas La Zarzuela, Madrid, Spain

Universidad Rey Juan Carlos, Madrid, Spain
e-mail: guillermo.plaza@salud.madrid.org

J. J. Navarro Sampedro
Ear, Nose and Throat Department, Hospital Universitario de Donostia,
Donostia-San Sebastián, Gipuzkoa, Spain

C. O'Connor Reina
Ear, Nose and Throat Department, Hospitales Quirónsalud Marbella and Campo de Gibraltar,
Cádiz, Spain

C. Rodríguez Izquierdo
Ear, Nose and Throat Department, Hospital Universitario de Fuenlabrada, Madrid, Spain

J. R. García Berrocal
Ear, Nose and Throat Department, Hospital Universitario Puerto de Hierro, Majadahonda,
Madrid, Spain

Universidad Autónoma de Madrid, Madrid, Spain

Third, the field of cochlear therapy, through cochlear regeneration and gene therapy, still in its beginnings, is without doubt the most promising to resolve ISSNHL in the near future.

New Drugs for the Inner Ear

After many years of having corticosteroids as the most common treatment of ISSNHL, at present, there are new drugs in development that hopefully in the next years will change treatment of pathology of the inner ear [4–11] (Table 1).

Dinh et al. [12] reviewed the factors that contribute to the loss of hair cells in the organ of Corti, ultimately to the cause of deafness: inflammatory processes, oxidative stress, mitochondrial damage and death of cell receptors and proteins. In essence, subjected to damage, the stria vascularis and the ligament spiral release TNF-alpha, which in turn stimulates many other cytokines and the mitogenic protein kinase chain activated (MAPK), leading to apoptosis cell via c-Jun N-terminal protein (JNK). These processes are the main target that sustain the mechanism of action of glucocorticoids, but also, they are the target of some new drugs (Fig. 1).

For instance, the JNK kinase cascade serves as target for a new drug, AM-111 (brimapitide; Auris Medical AG, Basel, Switzerland). It is a 31-amino acid cell-permeable peptide that acts as an inhibitor of the JNK stress kinase, having been shown to protect against cell death by extrinsic apoptosis, promoting hearing preservation [12]. In 2014, Suckfüll et al. [13] published a randomised clinical trial (RCT) on the efficacy and safety of AM-111 as primary treatment intratympanic of ISSNHL. They compared three groups: placebo, 0.4 mg/ml, or 2 mg/ml drug, through a single infiltration. Only for severe cases, with hearing worse than 60 dB, AM-111 at a dose of 0.4 mg/ml was more effective than placebo. Staecker et al. [14] also published a double-blind, randomised, placebo-controlled phase 3 with AM-111 in patients with ISSNHL with also a single treatment. Similarly, they found a clinically relevant and nominally significant treatment effect for AM-111 0.4 mg/

Table 1 Pharmacological novelties for pathology of the inner ear

Drug	Mechanism of action
AM-111 (brimapitide)	Inhibitor of the JNK stress kinase
N-Acetylcysteine (NAC)	Precursor of glutathione, reducing the production of ROS
Vitamins A, C and E	Antioxidants of various mechanisms
Ginkgo biloba Linn (Ginkgoaceae) leaves extract (GBE)	Scavenges oxygen free radicals, improves vascular microcirculation, and reduces blood viscosity
Etanercept, infliximab	Immunomodulators
Insulin-like growth factor-1 (IGF-1)	Important modulator of neurogenesis and hearing development, whose protective effect on hair cells has
Nerve growth factor (NGF)	Nerve cell growth regulator possessing dual biological functions

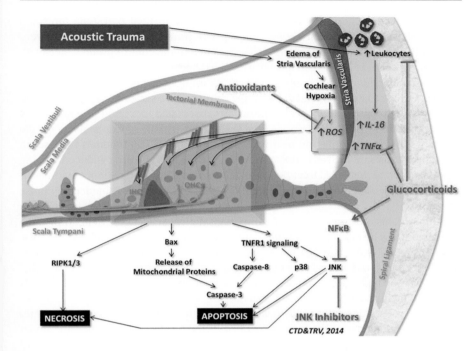

Fig. 1 New pharmacological therapies for pathology of the inner ear. Different noxas cause oedema of the stria vascularis, causing cochlear hypoxia, formation of free radicals (ROS) and stress oxidative. This produces the release of pro-inflammatory cytokines that affect the hair cells, such as TNF-alpha and IL-1beta, and prolonged activation of the JNK protein, promoting apoptosis. Glucocorticoids, antioxidants and inhibitors of the JNK protein (AM-111) work by altering some of these stress mechanisms. (Modified from Dinh et al. [12] https://creativecommons.org/licenses/by/4.0/)

ml in patients with profound ISSNHL. However, this treatment is not clinically available yet.

Antioxidants act through the protection of the glutathione pathway, decreasing free radicals and protecting from cell death, trying to preserve hearing [15]. Among them, N-acetylcysteine (NAC) is a precursor of glutathione, which is a critical antioxidant in the human body [16, 17]. Reactive oxygen species (ROS), as oxygen-containing radicals, can damage auditory hair cells by activating apoptotic cell death programmes [18], and NAC can reduce the production of ROS to protect hair cells in the inner ear from damage [19]. Thus, the mechanism of action of NAC in the treatment of ISSNHL is based on altering the oxidative status that contributes to cochlear injury [20, 21]. Pathak et al. [22] found that NAC also reduced TNF-alpha levels in patients with immune-mediated hearing loss. Sarafraz et al. [23] published an RCT applying NAC or dexamethasone transtympanically to prevent cisplatin-induced toxicity in patients, observing greater conservation of hearing with NAC. Bai et al. [24] also published an RCT comparing whether oral NAC improved the results of intratympanic dexamethasone as a salvage treatment of

ISSNHL. Overall, there was no statistical difference in final pure-tone threshold average (PTA) improvement between those two groups but the hearing recovery rates of the NAC group were much higher than that in the control group. Chen et al. [25] retrospectively compared primary ISSNHL cases treated with oral steroids alone or combined to NAC, finding similar PTA improvements, only better for NAC at 8 kHz. Kouka et al. [26] found in a large retrospective series of 793 patients that adding NAC to prednisolone was significantly associated to a good prognosis (OR 1.862; CI 1.200–2.887). Finally, Bai et al. [27] presented a meta-analysis on the effect of NAC in sensorineural hearing loss, including 1197 individuals from seven published studies on ISSNHL, noise-induced hearing loss and drug-induced hearing loss. They found that NAC treatment was linked with improved patient outcomes of hearing tests in cases of ISSNHL, but did not prevent hearing loss induced by noise or ototoxicity.

Antioxidants are considered to be important radical scavengers to neutralise the oxidative stress by enhancing cellular defences and then protect the cell membranes. Vitamins (A, C and E) are the major antioxidant vitamins. Each vitamin has a different mechanism of action, for example, vitamin A can reduce the concentration of singlet oxygen and repair damaged hair cells, vitamin E can reduce peroxyl radicals in the cell membrane, and vitamin C can detoxify free radicals in the aqueous phase. A recent systematic review [28] has shown that these vitamins can significantly improve the outcome of the management of ISSNHL [29–31]. Another line under study is the use of antioxidants acting through the A1 adenosine receptor which will reduce ROS and get less activity MAPK, and therefore, greater acoustic protection [32].

Ginkgo biloba Linn (Ginkgoaceae) leaves extract (GBE) is an active ingredient extracted from the dried leaves of Ginkgo biloba [33, 34], with the effects of promoting blood circulation and removing blood stasis, activating the collaterals to relieve pain, warming the lungs and relieving asthma, removing turbidity and reducing lipid. The main active ingredients contain ginkgolides and flavonoid glycosides, which can inhibit the formation of ear thrombus, scavenge oxygen-free radicals, improve vascular microcirculation and reduce blood viscosity [34–36]. It can effectively promote inner ear microcirculation, help patients recover from hearing dysfunction and accelerate the relief of tinnitus and vertigo, which exerts significant pharmacological activity on ISSNHL. GBE exerts significant antioxidant activity [37], which can improve the activity of superoxide dismutase [34], accelerate the scavenging of oxygen-free radicals caused by ischaemia and protect cell tissues. GBE also has vasodilator effect, can stimulate the production of endothelium-derived relaxing factor and prostacyclin, promote the relaxation of vascular smooth muscle, which could maintain good arteriovenous tension, and increase the blood flow in and around the injury spot [38]. GBE dilates the auricular arterioles, increases the blood flow of the inner ear, enhances the compensatory function of the inner ear, improves tissue metabolism, alleviates labyrinthine artery oedema and accelerates the disappearance of clinical symptoms. This has promoted many RCTs on the effect of GBE in ISSNHL, such as the one by Koo et al. [39] showing better results in speech discrimination scores when GBE was added to steroids. A large number of randomised controlled trials from Asia had been reviewed in two recent meta-analyses including 27 articles with a total of 2623 patients. Yuan et al. [40] revealed that the effects of GBE adjuvant therapy were superior to general treatment: total effective rate (RR = 1.22, 95% CI: 1.18–1.26), and the pure tone hearing threshold and hemorheology indexes after treatment were significantly improved compared to non-treatment. Si et al. [41] obtained very similar results including A total of 11 RCTs involving 1069 patients. However, the GRADE assessment indicated that the overall strength of evidence was not high. Further studies with high methodological quality and low risk of bias are needed to confirm the positive results.

Some of the immunomodulators (azathioprine, etanercept, infliximab, adalimumab, rituximab, etc.) used in immune-mediated disease of the inner ear could be used intratympanically to improve hearing loss [42–44]. Sharaf et al. [45] observed that etanercept was able to reverse the decreased cochlear flow induced by TNF-alpha. Dasli et al. [46] proposed etanercept to prevent cisplatin-induced toxicity in patients, with a single intraperoneal dose. Van Wijk et al. [47] used infliximab, an anti-TNF-alpha, transtympanically through a Microwick®, managing to reduce the dose of oral steroids and maintaining hearing gain.

Other authors have also tested the role of insulin-like growth factors (IGFs) in ISSNHL, the most used is IGF-1. It is a polypeptide of 70 amino acids with a molecular weight of 7649 Da and an important modulator of neurogenesis and hearing development, whose protective effect on hair cells has been extensively studied [48, 49]. Clinical studies have revealed that local IGF-1 administration to the round window niche via gelatin hydrogel can improve hearing levels in patients with sudden sensorineural hearing loss refractory to systemic steroids [50–52]. In 2010, Nakagawa et al. [50] presented a work on the IGF-1 applied intratympanically in a gelatin hydrogel as a single dose in patients with ISSNHL as rescue after failed systemic treatment, with promising results. Later, in 2012, Nakagawa et al. [51] presented the audiometric results after a single intratympanic dose of IGF-1 in hydrogel in 25 patients with ISSNHL after the failure of the systemic treatment, confirming the improvement with a mean of 12 dB (CI 6–18 dB), stabilised at 4 weeks of it. Subsequently, in 2016, Nakagawa et al. [52] published an RCT comparing a single dose of intratympanic IGF-1 in hydrogel with four intratympanic doses of dexamethasone (3.8 mg/ml) in 120 patients with ISSNHL after the failure of the systemic treatment. In both groups, there was improvement of >10 dB in >50% of patients, with no differences significant between them (66% vs. 57%). However, the average gain in dB was significantly higher with IGF-1. However, in terms of the size of delivered substances, the round window membrane (RWM) is more permeable to smaller substances [53]. As IGF-1 has a larger molecular weight than low molecular weight drugs, such as dexamethasone, several pharmacokinetics designs are currently developed to enhance the ability of IGF-1 to pass through the RWM and thus improve the therapeutic effect of IGF-1, such as ultrasound microbubbles [49, 54, 55].

Finally, ongoing research has demonstrated that exogenous nerve growth factor (NGF) can mitigate the damage caused by noise and ototoxic drugs to cochlear hair cells [56–58]. Han et al. [59] revealed that NGF plays a vital role in the differentiation of cochlear neural stem cells into functional neurons while reducing the ototoxicity of gentamicin. These findings suggest the potential for NGF in the treatment of hearing loss. NGF is known to be a nerve cell growth regulator possessing dual biological functions, acting on vegetative neurons and promoting the growth of processes. It plays a significant role in the regulation of development, regeneration of central and peripheral neurons, and the expression of functional characteristics. NGF has been widely utilised in research investigating the treatment of neurological diseases [60]. Liang et al. [61] showed that adding NGF to conventional treatment enhanced the audiometric improvement: the hearing recovery effective rate in the control group was 42.1%, while that of the experimental group reached 70.5%, with a statistically significant difference between the groups in a retrospective study.

Improvements in Pharmacokinetics of the Inner Ear

At the end of the twentieth century, we witnessed the introduction of intratympanic route for the administration of drugs to the inner ear (Fig. 2), having shown that this route is superior to systemic administration. Currently, the challenge is to improve the intratympanic delivery of drugs through the RWM to the inner ear [62], using

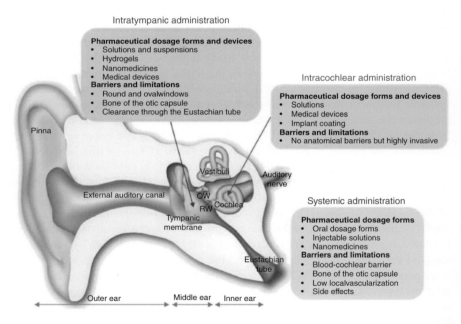

Fig. 2 Comparison between the routes of drug administration to the inner ear: systemic, intratympanic and intracochlear. (Taken from El Kechai et al. (2015) Reprinted with permission from: El Kechai N, Agnely F, Mamelle E, et al. Recent advances in local drug delivery to the inner ear. Int J Pharm. 2015; 494: 83-101)

facilitators or vehicles, as suspensions, hydrogels or nanoparticles [63–65], with the aim of increasing the diffusion, concentration and duration of drugs in the inner ear.

As facilitating agents, Borden et al. [66] proposed transporting intratympanic steroids with hyaluronic acid gel to facilitate its passage through the RWM in an experimental model; they achieved higher concentration in perilymph with this gel, which persisted up to 48 h after its administration. In humans, hyaluronic acid gel has been used with dexamethasone intratympanic in ISSNHL by Gouveris et al. [67, 68] and Selinova et al. [69]

Chandrasekhar et al. [70] compared the perilymph concentration reached after the administration of intratympanic injection of dexamethasone using three different facilitators: histamine, hyaluronic acid and dimethyl sulfoxide. They observed that the permeability was higher when histamine was used. Similarly, Creber et al. [71, 72] compared in guinea pigs the administration of dexamethasone, associated with histamine, hyaluronic acid or both. Taking perilymph measurements gradually from the base to the apex, and using immunohistochemistry to assess the distribution in the cochlea, they have shown higher concentrations of dexamethasone in the base of the cochlea, and a more uniform distribution when using hyaluronic acid.

Hydrogels have also been used to transport steroids intratympanically [73, 74]. They are composed of a water-soluble matrix in which the drug dissolves and allows its diffusion controlled [75, 76]. Hydrogels have been used in guinea pigs to facilitate intratympanic diffusion of dexamethasone and insulin-like growth factor (IGF-1) [50] and in humans to test its efficacy in ISSNHL [51, 52]. Honeder et al. [77] used hydrogel to administer intratympanically triamcinolone in guinea pigs, obtaining very good concentrations in perilymph. Lei et al. [78] evaluated the hearing outcome of dexamethasone sodium phosphate delivery to the round window niche by saturated gelatin sponge for refractory sudden sensorineural hearing loss in 20 patients. They showed it may be a simple and feasible way to treat refractory sudden sensorineural hearing loss with a risk of permanent tympanic membrane perforation.

Plontke et al. [79] used acid polymers poly-lactic-co-glycolic acid (PLGA) to release dexamethasone through the RWM in patients with ISSNHL after the failure of systemic treatment. The biodegradable drug delivery system was implanted in the RW niche. The PLGA matrix slowly degrades to lactic acid and glycolic acid, allowing controlled release drug delivery to the inner ear. They have recently shown its efficacy in the release of steroids obtaining promising results, including 6 out of 15 patients /40% reaching serviceable hearing [80] (Fig. 3). More recently, Dai et al. [81] developed a chitosan hydrogel thermally biodegradable, with better release of interferon in the cochlea of guinea pigs.

Nanomedicine provides new strategies for the diffusion of drugs into the inner ear by nanoparticles of different materials [63, 64], as chitosan, polyglycolic acid, magnetic nano-carriers, liposomes, etc. [9, 82–86], and for different purposes, such as investigating the passage of toxins to the inner ear or to transport drugs, growth factors or genes into the ear internal. Thus, for example, polymeric nanoparticles based on smart amphiphilic copolymers have been used to transport and release in a controlled manner dexamethasone into the inner ear with the aim of protecting

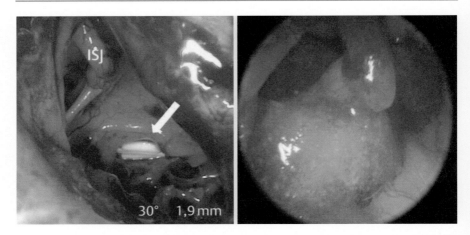

Fig. 3 Particles of gels or polymers as drug vehicles for the inner ear in a round window. (Modified from Plontke (2017). https://creativecommons.org/licenses/by/4.0/)

Table 2 Advantages and disadvantages of the intratmpanic or intracochlear route [6, 88]

	Intratympanic	Intracochlear
Pros	Easy access	Dose control
	Minimal risk of hearing loss	Greater bioavailability
	Minimal surgical trauma	Less loss of drug
	Local anaesthesia	Ideal associated with cochlear implantation
Cons	Worse bioavailability	Hard access
	Dose control variable	General anaesthesia
	Variable patency due to round window fibrosis	Hearing compromised

against the ototoxic effect of cisplatin [84]. For a long time, it has been considered that the passage of these nanoparticles to the inner ear was exclusively through the RWM. However, Ding et al. [87] presented an interesting work on the passage of chitosan nanoparticles to the vestibule through the oval window. According to this study, nanoparticles penetrate more through the oval window than through the round.

Finally, the development of the intracochlear pathway has been linked to the insertion of cochlear implants that release drugs or substances, once inserted in the cochlea itself during cochlear implantation [6, 88, 89] (Table 2). In the future, small intracochlear infusion pumps through a mini-cochleostomy may be the solution to preserve the cochlea. Lyu et al. [90] compared the distribution into the inner ear of dexamethasone administered in guinea pigs by systemic, intratympanic or intracochlear route. Through this last route, the concentration of hearing recovery was greater, while the release of cytokines inflammatory (IL-1, IL-6, TNF-alpha and NOS2) and histological changes were minor.

Cochlear Regeneration and Gene Therapy

The organ of Corti is primarily responsible for the auditory sensation and corresponds to a highly organised and differentiated epithelium [91]. This organ contains sensory cells or ciliates (CC) and support cells (SC) of different types. We only have 15,000 hair cells per cochlea. Both cell types play roles fundamental and interdependent. However, most hearing disorders are related to irreversible damage of the CC, making the CS more resistant to damage [92].

When moderate damage is present, CCs are expelled from the neurosensory epithelium and the left spaces are replaced by extensions of nearby CS to maintain their electrochemical integrity and survival. For this reason, CS are a possible therapeutic target of regenerative therapies. However, when severe or prolonged damage is present, the neurosensory epithelium is replaced by a squamous epithelium, compromising the health of the entire inner ear, its connections with the central nervous system and the potential benefits of future treatments [93]. Unlike Reissner's membrane, which can be repaired after suffering damage, the mammalian cochlea has lost the ability to spontaneous regeneration. In contrast, lower vertebrates (fish, batrachians and reptiles) do have a permanent renewal of the hair cell population under normal conditions and also after an injury. This leads to an important field of investigations in the near future [94–98].

Since 2003 it has been known that there are pluripotent stem cells in the mouse utricle and that can differentiate into hair cells [99]. However, it has been seen that the number of stem cells present in the adult cochlea of mammals is much smaller. For this reason, manipulation was attempted to make somatic cells become stem cells. These induced pluripotent stem cells to differentiate into hair cells, creating thus a newly formed inner ear [100]. Another therapeutic option is cell transplantation. Marrow-derived mesenchymal stem bone of the patient for its later development in hair cells [101]. This would be the way for an eventual cochlear transplant in the future.

Gene therapy tries to correct genetic errors that cause disease, and this has been also directed to the inner ear [102–105]. To achieve this, one of the most frequent ways consists of infecting the patient with the gene suitable using a virus. Many of these genes are altered in patients with hearing loss of genetic cause (e.g. TBX1 and Sd. DiGeorge). However, some of them are also expressed in the adult inner ear, and although their function is not fully known, they are often used as markers of certain cells of the organ of Corti. These genes encode various products: secreted or membrane proteins (e.g. Notch/Delta-Jag1y2 and Fgfr3/Fgf8), factors transcription (e.g. Atoh1, Hes1, Hes5 and Tbx1) and cell cycle regulators (pRb and p27Kip1). The manipulation of the expression of some of these genes in the organ of Corti has produced proliferation cell and new hair cells, demonstrating that there is regenerative potential.

Another line of research would be the introduction or modification of certain genes responsible for sensorineural hearing loss in specific diseases [106, 107]. This method has already been used in some hearing loss congenital such as in Usher syndrome [108]. This therapy has a great potential, but still is very limited for acquired sensorineural hearing loss as ISSNHL [109, 110].

Conclusions

So far, there is no definitive treatment for ISSNHL. Several new therapies have been developed, from new drugs still under evaluation to modern pharmacokinetic designs to enhance diffusion into the inner ear. In the next future, new treatments designed to regenerate inner ear hair cells and gene therapy will be key to helping patients with ISSNHL.

References

1. Rauch SD. Clinical practice. Idiopathic sudden sensorineural hearing loss. N Engl J Med. 2008;359:833–40.
2. Herrera M, García Berrocal JR, García Arumí A, et al. Update on consensus on diagnosis and treatment of idiopathic sudden sensorineural hearing loss. Acta Otorrinolaringol Esp (Engl Ed). 2019;70:290–300.
3. Chandrasekhar SS, Tsai Do BS, Schwartz SR, et al. Clinical practice guideline: sudden hearing loss (update). Otolaryngol Head Neck Surg. 2019;161(Suppl. 1):S1–S45.
4. Yamada S, Kita J, Shinmura D, Nakamura Y, et al. Update on findings about sudden sensorineural hearing loss and insight into its pathogenesis. J Clin Med. 2022;11:6387.
5. Plaza MG. Novedades terapéuticas en sordera súbita idiopática. In: Plaza G, editor. Sordera súbita: diagnóstico y tratamiento. Madrid: Ergon; 2018. p. 259–67.
6. Rivera T, Sanz L, Camarero G, Varela-Nieto I. Drug delivery to the inner ear: strategies and their therapeutic implications for sensorineural hearing loss. Curr Drug Deliv. 2012;9:231–42.
7. Bird PA, Bergin MJ. Pharmacological issues in hearing rehabilitation. Adv Otorhinolaryngol. 2018;81:114–22.
8. Bodmer D. An update on drug design strategies to prevent acquired sensorineural hearing loss. Expert Opin Drug Discov. 2017;12:1161–7.
9. El Kechai N, Agnely F, Mamelle E, et al. Recent advances in local drug delivery to the inner ear. Int J Pharm. 2015;494:83–101.
10. Lalwani AK, Qian ZJ, McGuire JF. Pharmacologic and molecular therapies of the cochlear and vestibular labyrinths. In: Flint WP, Haughey BH, Lund VJ, et al., editors. Cummings otolaryngology head and neck surgery. 6th ed. Philadelphia: Elsevier Saunders; 2015. p. 2383–99.
11. Musazzi UM, Franzé S, Cilurzo F. Innovative pharmaceutical approaches for the management of inner ear disorders. Drug Deliv Transl Res. 2018;8:436–49.
12. Dinh CT, Goncalves S, Bas E, et al. Molecular regulation of auditory hair cell death and approaches to protect sensory receptor cells and/or stimulate repair following acoustic trauma. Front Cell Neurosci. 2015;9:96.
13. Suckfüll M, Lisowska G, Domka W, et al. Efficacy and safety of AM-111 in the treatment of acute sensorineural hearing loss: a double-blind, randomized, placebo-controlled phase II study. Otol Neurotol. 2014;35:1317–26.
14. Staecker H, Jokovic G, Karpishchenko S, et al. Efficacy and safety of AM-111 in the treatment of acute unilateral sudden deafness-a double-blind, randomized, placebo-controlled phase 3 study. Otol Neurotol. 2019;40:584–94.
15. Goncalves S, Perez E, Bas E, et al. Trauma, inflammation, cochlear implantation induced hearing loss and otoprotective strategies to limit hair cell death and hearing loss. In: Ramkumar V, Rybak LP, editors. Inflammatory mechanisms in mediating hearing loss. Cham, Switzerland: Springer International Publishing AG, part of Springer Nature; 2018. p. 165–87.
16. Duan M, Qiu J, Laurell G, et al. Dose and time-dependent protection of the antioxidant N-L-acetylcysteine against impulse noise trauma. Hear Res. 2004;192:1–9.

17. Lin CY, Wu JL, Shih TS, et al. N-Acetyl-cysteine against noise-induced temporary threshold shift in male workers. Hear Res. 2010;269:42–7.
18. Kamogashira T, Fujimoto C, Yamasoba T. Reactive oxygen species, apoptosis, and mitochondrial dysfunction in hearing loss. Biomed Res Int. 2015;2015:617207.
19. Cotgreave IA. N-acetylcysteine: pharmacological considerations and experimental and clinical applications. Adv Pharmacol. 1997;38:205–27.
20. Angeli SI, Abi-Hachem RN, Vivero RJ, et al. L-N-Acetylcysteine treatment is associated with improved hearing outcome in sudden idiopathic sensorineural hearing loss. Acta Otolaryngol. 2012;132:369–76.
21. Chen CH, Young YH. N-acetylcysteine as a single therapy for sudden deafness. Acta Otolaryngol. 2017;137:58–62.
22. Pathak S, Stern C, Vambutas A. N-Acetylcysteine attenuates tumor necrosis factor alpha levels in autoimmune inner ear disease patients. Immunol Res. 2015;63:236–45.
23. Sarafraz Z, Ahmadi A, Daneshi A. Transtympanic injections of n-acetylcysteine and dexamethasone for prevention of cisplatin-induced ototoxicity: double blind randomized clinical trial. Int Tinnitus J. 2018;22:40–5.
24. Bai X, Chen S, Xu K, et al. N-Acetylcysteine combined with dexamethasone treatment improves sudden sensorineural hearing loss and attenuates hair cell death caused by ROS stress. Front Cell Dev Biol. 2021;9:659486.
25. Chen SL, Ho CY, Chin SC. Effects of oral N-acetylcysteine combined with oral prednisolone on idiopathic sudden sensorineural hearing loss. Medicine (Baltimore). 2022;101:e29792.
26. Kouka M, Bevern N, Bitter J, Guntinas-Lichius O. N-Acetylcysteine combined with prednisolone treatment shows better hearing outcome than treatment with prednisolone alone for patients with idiopathic sudden sensorineural hearing loss: a retrospective observational study. Eur Arch Otorhinolaryngol. 2024;281(1):107–16.
27. Bai X, Wang M, Niu X, et al. Effect of N-acetyl-cysteine treatment on sensorineural hearing loss: a meta-analysis. World J Otorhinolaryngol Head Neck Surg. 2022;8:205–12.
28. Ibrahim I, Zeitouni A, da Silva SD. Effect of antioxidant vitamins as adjuvant therapy for sudden sensorineural hearing loss: Systematic review study. Audiol Neurootol. 2018;23:1–7.
29. Joachims HZ, Segal J, Golz A, et al. Antioxidants in treatment of idiopathic sudden hearing loss. Otol Neurotol. 2003;24:572–5.
30. Hatano M, Uramoto N, Okabe Y, et al. Vitamin E and vitamin C in the treatment of idiopathic sudden sensorineural hearing loss. Acta Otolaryngol. 2008;128:116–21.
31. Kaya H, Ko AK, Sayın İ, et al. Vitamins A, C, and E and selenium in the treatment of idiopathic sudden sensorineural hearing loss. Eur Arch Otorrinolaringol. 2015;272:1119–25.
32. Sheth S, Mukherjea D, Rybak LP, Ramkumar V. The contribution of anti-oxidant and anti-inflammatory functions of adenosine A1 receptor in mediating otoprotection. In: Ramkumar V, Rybak LP, editors. Inflammatory mechanisms in mediating hearing loss. Cham, Switzerland: Springer International Publishing AG, part of Springer Nature; 2018. p. 149–64.
33. Yang Y, Zhou B, Zhao WJ. Ginkgo biloba leaves history: a model of research and development for Chinese material medical/phytomedicine. Chin Herbal Med. 2016;47:2579–91.
34. Barth SW, Lehner MD, Dietz GPH, Schulze H. Pharmacologic treatments in preclinical tinnitus models with special focus on Ginkgo biloba leaf extract EGb 761. Mol Cell Neurosci. 2021;116:103669.
35. Wang X. Observation on the efficacy of Ginkgo biloba extract injection in the treatment of sudden deafness. Health Care Guide. 2017;48:161.
36. Wang L, Li WT. Clinical observation of 61 cases of sudden deafness treated with Ginkgo biloba extract. Chin J Pract Nerv Dis. 2008;11:129–30.
37. Singh SK, Srivastav S, Castellani RJ, Plascencia-Villa G, Perry G. Neuroprotective and antioxidant effect of Ginkgo biloba extract against AD and other neurological disorders. Neurotherapeutics. 2019;16:666–74.
38. Tian J, Liu Y, Chen K. Ginkgo biloba extract in vascular protection: molecular mechanisms and clinical applications. Curr Vasc Pharmacol. 2017;15:532–48.

39. Koo JW, Chang MY, Yun SC, et al. The efficacy and safety of systemic injection of Ginkgo biloba extract, EGb761, in idiopathic sudden sensorineural hearing loss: a randomized placebo-controlled clinical trial. Eur Arch Otorrinolaringol. 2016;273:2433–41.
40. Si X, Yu Z, Ren X, et al. Efficacy and safety of standardized Ginkgo biloba L. leaves extract as an adjuvant therapy for sudden sensorineural hearing loss: a systematic review and meta-analysis. J Ethnopharmacol. 2022;282:114587.
41. Yuan C, Zhang H, Sun C, Zhang K. Efficacy and safety of Ginkgo bilobaextract as an adjuvant in the treatment of Chinese patients with sudden hearing loss: a meta-analysis. Pharm Biol. 2023;61:610–20.
42. Okano T. Immune system of the inner ear as a novel therapeutic target for sensorineural hearing loss. Front Pharmacol. 2014;5:205.
43. Windsor AM, Ruckenstein MJ. Anti-inflammatory therapies for sensorineural hearing loss. In: Ramkumar V, Rybak LP, editors. Inflammatory mechanisms in mediating hearing loss. Cham, Switzerland: Springer International Publishing AG, part of Springer Nature; 2018. p. 189–210.
44. Lobo Duro DR. Tesis doctoral: Terapias biológicas en la enfermedad inmunomediada del oído interno. In: Estudio clínico-experimental con etanercept. Madrid: Universidad Autónoma de Madrid; 2013.
45. Sharaf K, Ihler F, Bertlich M, et al. Tumor necrosis factor-induced decrease of cochlear blood flow can be reversed by etanercept or JTE-013. Otol Neurotol. 2016;37:e203–8.
46. Dasli S, Topdag M, Mutlu A, et al. Prophylactic etanercept treatment in cisplatin ototoxicity. Eur Arch Otorrinolaringol. 2017;274:3577–83.
47. Van Wijk F, Staecker H, Keithley E, Lefebvre PP. Local perfusion of the tumor necrosis factor alpha blocker infliximab to the inner ear improves autoimmune neurosensory hearing loss. Audiol Neurootol. 2006;11:357–65.
48. Murillo-Cuesta S, Rodríguez-de la Rosa L, Cediel R, aI. The role of insulin-like growth factor-I in the physiopathology of hearing. Front Mol Neurosci. 2011;4:11.
49. Yamahara K, Yamamoto N, Nakagawa T, Ito J. Insulin-like growth factor 1: a novel treatment for the protection or regeneration of cochlear hair cells. Hear Res. 2015;330:2–9.
50. Nakagawa T, Sakamoto T, Hiraumi H, et al. Topical insulin-like growth factor 1 treatment using gelatin hydrogels for glucocorticoid-resistant sudden sensorineural hearing loss: a prospective clinical trial. BMC Med. 2010;8:76.
51. Nakagawa T, Ogino-Nishimura E, Hiraumi H, et al. Audiometric outcomes of topical IGF1 treatment for sudden deafness refractory to systemic steroids. Otol Neurotol. 2012;33:941–6.
52. Nakagawa T, Kumakawa K, Usami S, et al. A randomized controlled clinical trial of topical insulin-like growth factor-1 therapy for sudden deafness refractory to systemic corticosteroid treatment. BMC Med. 2014;12:219.
53. Juhn SK, Hamaguchi Y, Goycoolea M. Review of round window membrane permeability. Acta Otolaryngol. 1989;105(Suppl. 457):43–8.
54. Yamamoto N, Nakagawa T, Ito J. Application of insulin-like growth factor-1 in the treatment of inner ear disorders. Front Pharmacol. 2014;5:208.
55. Lin YC, Lin YY, Chen HC, et al. Ultrasound microbubbles enhance the efficacy of insulin-like growth factor-1 therapy for the treatment of noise-induced hearing loss. Molecules. 2021;26:3626.
56. Shoji F, Miller AL, Mitchell A, et al. Differential protective effects of neurotrophins in the attenuation of noise-induced hair cell loss. Hear Res. 2000;146:134–42.
57. Shah SB, Gladstone HB, Williams H, et al. An extended study: protective effects of nerve growth factor in neomycin-induced auditory neural degeneration. Am J Otol. 1995;163:310–4.
58. Zhai SQ, Yu N, Zhu YH, et al. Clinical efficacy of nerve growth factor in the treatment of blast-induced hearing loss: a pilot study. Eur Rev Med Pharmacol Sci. 2015;19:3146–51.
59. Han Z, Wang CP, Cong N, et al. Therapeutic value of nerve growth factor in promoting neural stem cell survival and differentiation and protecting against neuronal hearing loss. Mol Cell Biochem. 2017;428:149–59.
60. Wang SF, Zhang L, Zhang WW, et al. Mouse nerve growth factor for treatment of sudden deafness. Chin J Otol. 2016;14:223–8.

61. Liang Z, Gao M, Jia H, et al. Analysis of clinical efficacy and influencing factors of Nerve Growth Factor (NGF) treatment for sudden sensorineural hearing loss. Ear Nose Throat J. 2023:1455613231181711.
62. Nomura Y. Otological significance of the round window. Adv Otorhinolaryngol. 1984;33:66–72.
63. McCall AA, Swan EE, Borenstein JT, et al. Drug delivery for treatment of inner ear disease: current state of knowledge. Ear Hear. 2010;31:156–65.
64. Roy S, Glueckert R, Johnston AH, et al. Strategies for drug delivery to the human inner ear by multifunctional nanoparticles. Nanomedicine (Lond). 2012;7:55–63.
65. Swan EE, Mescher MJ, Sewell WF, et al. Inner ear drug delivery for auditory applications. Adv Drug Deliv Rev. 2008;60:1583–99.
66. Borden RC, Saunders JE, Berryhill WE, et al. Hyaluronic acid hydrogel sustains the delivery of dexamethasone across the round window membrane. Audiol Neurootol. 2011;16:1–11.
67. Gouveris H, Selivanova O, Mann W. Intratympanic dexamethasone with hyaluronic acid in the treatment of idiopathic sudden sensorineural hearing loss after failure of intravenous steroid and vasoactive therapy. Eur Arch Otorrinolaringol. 2005;262:131–4.
68. Gouveris H, Schuler-Schmidt W, Mewes T, Mann W. Intratympanic dexamethasone/hyaluronic acid mix as an adjunct to intravenous steroid and vasoactive treatment in patients with severe idiopathic sudden sensorineural hearing loss. Otol Neurotol. 2011;32:756–60.
69. Selivanova OA, Gouveris H, Victor A, et al. Intratympanic dexamethasone and hyaluronic acid in patients with low-frequency and Ménière's-associated sudden sensorineural hearing loss. Otol Neurotol. 2005;26:890–5.
70. Chandrasekhar SS, Rubinstein RY, Kwartler JA, et al. Dexamethasone pharmacokinetics in the inner ear: comparison of route of administration and use of facilitating agents. Otolaryngol Head Neck Surg. 2000;122:521–8.
71. Creber NJ, Eastwood HT, Hampson AJ, et al. A comparison of cochlear distribution and glucocorticoid receptor activation in local and systemic dexamethasone drug delivery regimes. Hear Res. 2018;368:75–85.
72. Creber NJ, Eastwood HT, Hampson AJ, et al. Adjuvant agents enhance round window membrane permeability to dexamethasone and modulate basal to apical cochlear gradients. Eur J Pharm Sci. 2019;126:69–81.
73. Sakamoto T, Nakagawa T, Horie RT, et al. Inner ear drug delivery system from the clinical point of view. Acta Otolaryngol Suppl. 2010;130(Suppl. 563):101–4.
74. Murillo-Cuesta S, Vallecillo N, Cediel R, et al. A comparative study of drug delivery methods targeted to the mouse inner ear: bullostomy versus transtympanic injection. J Vis Exp. 2017;(121):e54951. https://doi.org/10.3791/54951.
75. Lee KY, Nakagawa T, Okano T, et al. Novel therapy for hearing loss: delivery of insulin-like growth factor 1 to the cochlea using gelatin hydrogel. Otol Neurotol. 2007;28:976–81.
76. Paulson DP, Abuzeid W, Jiang H, et al. A novel controlled local drug delivery system for inner ear disease. Laryngoscope. 2008;118:706–11.
77. Honeder C, Engleder E, Schöpper H, et al. Sustained release of triamcinolone acetonide from an intratympanically applied hydrogel designed for the delivery of high glucocorticoid doses. Audiol Neurootol. 2014;19:193–202.
78. Lei X, Yin X, Hu L, et al. Delivery of dexamethasone to the round window niche by saturated gelatin sponge for refractory sudden sensorineural hearing loss: a preliminary study. Otol Neurotol. 2023;44:e63–7.
79. Plontke SK, Glien A, Rahne T, et al. Controlled release dexamethasone implants in the round window niche for salvage treatment of idiopathic sudden sensorineural hearing loss. Otol Neurotol. 2014;35:1168–71.
80. Plontke SK, Liebau A, Lehner E, et al. Safety and audiological outcome in a case series of tertiary therapy of sudden hearing loss with a biodegradable drug delivery implant for controlled release of dexamethasone to the inner ear. Front Neurosci. 2022;16:892777.

81. Dai J, Long W, Liang Z, et al. A novel vehicle for local protein delivery to the inner ear: injectable and biodegradable thermosensitive hydrogel loaded with PLGA nanoparticles. Drug Dev Ind Pharm. 2018;44:89–98.
82. El Kechai N, Mamelle E, Nguyen Y, et al. Hyaluronic acid liposomal gel sustains delivery of a corticoid to the inner ear. J Control Release. 2016;226:248–57.
83. Pyykkö I, Zou J, Schrott-Fischer A, et al. An overview of nanoparticle based delivery for treatment of inner ear disorders. Methods Mol Biol. 2016;1427:363–415.
84. Yang KJ, Son J, Jung SY, et al. Optimized phospholipid-based nanoparticles for inner ear drug delivery and therapy. Biomaterials. 2018;171:133–43.
85. Martín-Saldaña S, Palao-Suay R, Aguilar MR, Ramírez-Camacho R, San Román J. Polymeric nanoparticles loaded with dexamethasone or α-tocopheryl succinate to prevent cisplatin-induced ototoxicity. Acta Biomater. 2017;53:199–210.
86. Barbara M, Margani V, Covelli E, et al. The use of nanoparticles in otoprotection. Front Neurol. 2022;13:912647.
87. Ding S, Xie S, Chen W, et al. Is oval window transport a royal gate for nanoparticle delivery to vestibule in the inner ear? Eur J Pharm Sci. 2019;126:11–22.
88. Ayoob AM, Borenstein JT. The role of intracochlear drug delivery devices in the management of inner ear disease. Expert Opin Drug Deliv. 2015;12:465–79.
89. Chin OY, Diaz RC. State-of-the-art methods in clinical intracochlear drug delivery. Curr Opin Otolaryngol Head Neck Surg. 2019;27:381–6.
90. Lyu AR, Kim DH, Lee SH, et al. Effects of dexamethasone on intracochlear inflammation and residual hearing after cochleostomy: a comparison of administration routes. PLoS One. 2018;13:e0195230.
91. Rybak LP. The cochlea. In: Ramkumar V, Rybak LP, editors. Inflammatory mechanisms in mediating hearing loss. Cham, Switzerland: Springer International Publishing AG, part of Springer Nature; 2018. p. 1–13.
92. Maass JC, Hanuch F, Ormazábald M. Avances en regeneración auditiva. Estado actual y perspectivas futuras. Rev Méd Clín Condes. 2016;27:812–8.
93. Youm I, Li W. Cochlear hair cell regeneration: an emerging opportunity to cure noise-induced sensorineural hearing loss. Drug Discov Today. 2018;23:1564–9.
94. Revuelta M, Santaolalla F, Arteaga O, et al. Recent advances in cochlear hair cell regeneration—a promising opportunity for the treatment of age-related hearing loss. Ageing Res Rev. 2017;36:149–55.
95. Mittal R, Nguyen D, Patel AP, et al. Recent advancements in the regeneration of auditory hair cells and hearing restoration. Front Mol Neurosci. 2017;10:236.
96. Schilder AGM, Su MP, Blackshaw H, et al. Hearing protection, restoration, and regeneration: an overview of emerging therapeutics for inner ear and central hearing disorders. Otol Neurotol. 2019;40:559–70.
97. Kelleci K, Golebetmaz E. Regenerative therapy approaches and encountered problems in sensorineural hearing loss. Curr Stem Cell Res Ther. 2023;18:186–201.
98. Matsunaga M, Nakagawa T. Future pharmacotherapy for sensorineural hearing loss by protection and regeneration of auditory hair cells. Pharmaceutics. 2023;15:777.
99. Ibekwe TS, Ramma L, Chindo BA. Potential roles of stem cells in the management of sensorineural hearing loss. J Laryngol Otol. 2012;126:653–7.
100. Simoni E, Orsini G, Chicca M, et al. Regenerative medicine in hearing recovery. Cytotherapy. 2017;19:909–15.
101. Takeda H, Dondzillo A, Randall JA, Gubbels SP. Challenges in cell-based therapies for the treatment of hearing loss. Trends Neurosci. 2018;41:823–37.
102. Lee MY, Park YH. Potential of gene and cell therapy for inner ear hair cells. Biomed Res Int. 2018;2018:8137614.
103. Jones M, Kovacevic B, Ionescu CM, et al. The applications of targeted delivery for gene therapies in hearing loss. J Drug Target. 2023;31:585–95.
104. Wang J, Zheng J, Wang H, et al. Gene therapy: an emerging therapy for hair cells regeneration in the cochlea. Front Neurosci. 2023;17:1177791.

105. Lahlou G, Calvet C, Giorgi M, et al. Towards the clinical application of gene therapy for genetic inner ear diseases. J Clin Med. 2023;12:1046.
106. Yoon JY, Yang KJ, Park SN, et al. The effect of dexamethasone/cell-penetrating peptide nanoparticles on gene delivery for inner ear therapy. Int J Nanomed. 2016;11:6123–34.
107. Zhang W, Kim SM, Wang W, et al. Cochlear gene therapy for sensorineural hearing loss: current status and major remaining hurdles for translational success. Front Mol Neurosci. 2018;11:221.
108. Pan B, Askew C, Galvin A, et al. Gene therapy restores auditory and vestibular function in a mouse model of Usher syndrome type 1c. Nat Biotechnol. 2017;35:264–72.
109. Kanzaki S. Gene delivery into the inner ear and its clinical implications for hearing and balance. Molecules. 2018;23:2507.
110. Rzepakowska A, Borowy A, Siedlecki E, Wolszczak M, Radomska K. Contemporary directions in the therapy of sensory hearing loss. Otolaryngol Pol. 2024;78(4):29–38.